PERIPHERAL NERVE BLOCKS

In Emergency Medicine and Urgent Care

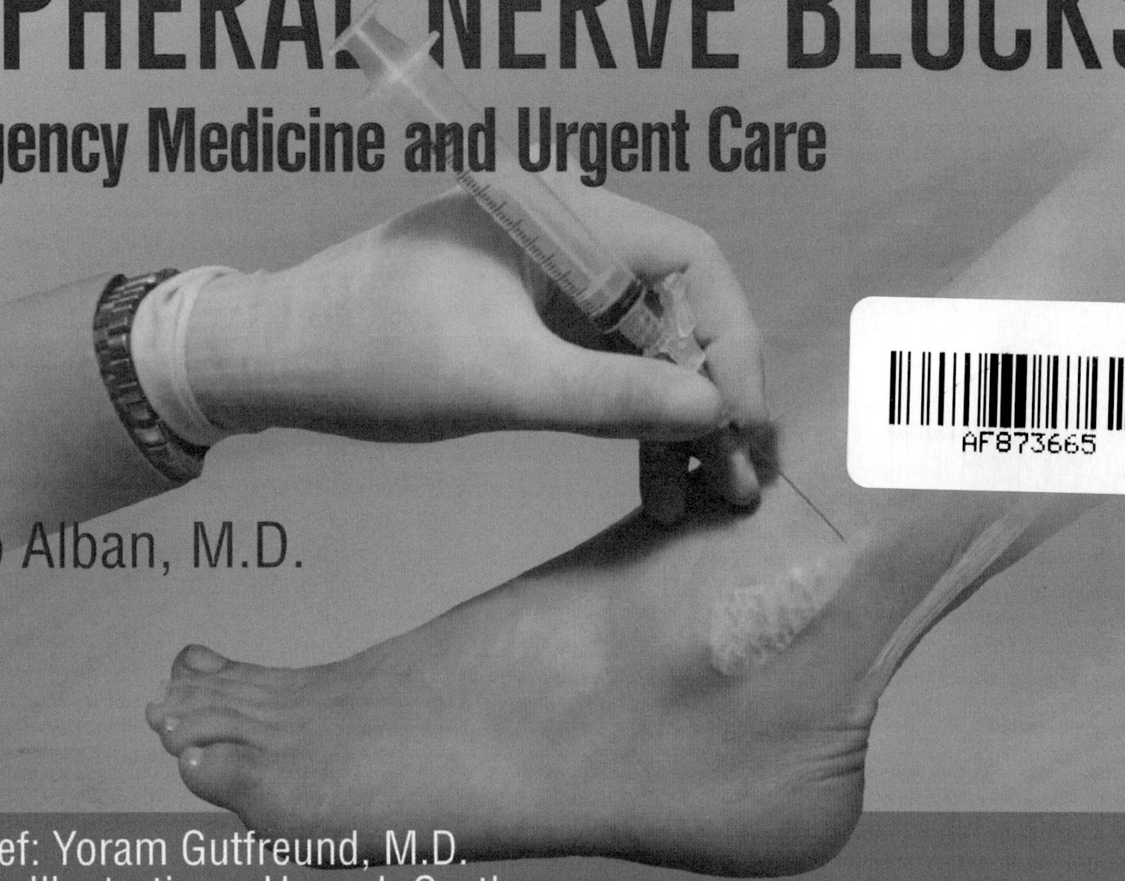

By Alvaro Alban, M.D.

Editor in Chief: Yoram Gutfreund, M.D.
Photography, Illustrations: Hannah Grotbo

Peripheral Nerve Blocks In Emergency Medicine And Urgent Care
Author: Alvaro Alban, M.D.
Editor In-Cheif: Yoram Gutfreund, M.D.
Illustrations & Photography: Hannah Grotbo
Revised Layout & Cover: Nicole Fuster

First Edition

ISBN: 978-0-578-92197-6

Printed and bound in the USA

TABLE OF CONTENTS

FOREWORD

This handbook is organized in order of importance from the most commonly used peripheral nerve blocks to the least commonly used in emergency medicine and urgent care.

What is a peripheral nerve block? A peripheral nerve block treats pain transmitted via sensory nerves to the spinal cord. The block involves injecting local anesthetic as close as possible to the nerve carrying the pain signal. It is primarily used to relieve pain at the site of injury, especially before performing a clinical procedure.

How to use this pocket manual

Read the first few pages and understand what this abbreviated pocket manual covers and what it doesn't cover. When you encounter a patient that requires local anesthesia, flip through the sensory distribution pictures and locate the section that addresses the area you need to block.

First, understand what sensory area of the body is covered by the nerve you are blocking. Then go to the procedure section and read it carefully, reviewing all the pictures and diagrams pertaining to the block you are about to perform.

The procedure sections should serve as a review of the peripheral nerve block and not as a primary source. The alternative is to look through the table of contents and find the block you are looking for by name and to turn to that page directly.

Disclaimer

This guide is for physicians, mid-level providers, residents, and supervised medical students who want a practical guide for the most common and most useful peripheral nerve blocks. This book does not replace a formal textbook of peripheral anesthesia, nor does it replace an anatomy text. It is an abbreviated guide that requires formal training in human anatomy, pharmacology, and clinical experience in the use of needles, proper sterile technique and clinical safety precautions.

Note

The equipment photographed in this manual is for illustration purposes and should not indicate any specific endorsement.

Layout of manual

I've started most sections with illustrations of sensory nerve distributions. Then the specific nerve block is discussed along with pictures depicting landmarks on human subjects. Certain drawings are included where pictures will not suffice. In some cases, I've included details about the anatomy because I believe that knowing the names and locations of landmark tendons, muscles, and arterial pulses is what will give you the confidence to carry out these procedures. In cases where there are multiple approaches for performing a block, I've chosen to include only my favorite approach, the one I presently use in clinical practice.

General indications for peripheral nerve blocks and some specifics

The blocks presented in this manual are used primarily for anesthesia during laceration repair, debridement of tissue, other trauma to the affected part, and neuralgia from various causes. They are also important in providing anesthesia for a variety of clinical procedures in emergency medicine and urgent care such as incision and drainage of abscess, foreign body removal, and any other procedure that requires a painful intervention. Blocks that involve the face and scalp are particularly useful for pain management related to shingles and neuralgia. The femoral nerve block presented here is used to manage pain from a femur fracture. The intercostal block described is useful for pain due to a rib fracture but can also be used for pain complaints after a nephrectomy or any other surgical intervention that requires iatrogenic rib injury. Recently, the occipital nerve blocks have been described for the treatment of tension headaches.

Why use a nerve block rather than local infiltration

Local injections directly into injury sites create swelling of tissues which makes suturing more difficult and leads to less-than-ideal cosmetic results. With local infiltration, the wound can become distorted and adversely affect the approximation of wound margins. Further, the swelling creates increased, unwanted wound tension. There are certain areas where injecting large volumes of anesthetic can be quite painful due to space confinements, such as the fingers, toes, nose, or penis. If larger areas of the body require anesthesia, local injections of anesthetic may result in too much anesthetic being used and concerns of toxicity could become an issue. Peripheral nerve blocks for these larger areas could be done with much less injected volume. Finally, patients are squeamish about injecting right into the injury they've just suffered.

A note on local infiltration

For areas of the body not covered by the nerve blocks in this manual, local infiltration is often indicated. When performing local infiltration, inject anesthetic into the wound edge as opposed to the skin. This results in less pain. Ideal needle for blocking: The 25-ga needle is appropriate for all of the blocks discussed in this manual. In some cases you may need a 25-ga needle that is at least 3cm long.

Occasionally these are not available in all emergency departments or urgent care centers. It is important to request that hospital administration or the urgent care proprietor(s) make available the correct size needles at all times. Using a thinner needle is appropriate because it lowers the incidence of nerve injury and decreases the pain of the injection. Otherwise, do not use a needle with a greater caliber than 25-ga.

A note on sterile technique and aspiration: At all times you must use sterile technique for the procedures discussed here. This includes but is not limited to using sterile gloves, gowns, caps, masks, and needles. Further, the area injected must first be properly wiped with alcohol. When you withdraw anesthesia from a bottle to a syringe always use sterile precautions. In order to avoid redundancy these important sterile techniques are not included in each section of this manual. Before injecting anesthesia while performing a block, aspirate to make sure the needle is not cannulated in an artery or a vein.

If you withdraw blood from aspiration, reposition the needle. Again this important step is not included in many of the nerve block sections below. Eliciting paresthesia with the needle upon insertion: While performing any of the nerve blocks described in this manual, if you elicit paresthesia during the insertion of your needle, this is good and bad. It's bad because injecting anesthetic itself into the nerve or moving the needle haphazardly at this point could cause nerve injury. It's good because you have found the exact location where anesthesia should be deposited. When you elicit paresthesia, do not worry. Simply pull back about one millimeter and inject your anesthetic.

What anesthetic should I use and what are the maximum dosages

Use lidocaine 1% - 2% for most of the blocks covered in this manual. You could use epinephrine with lidocaine for all the blocks except for digits, toes, ears, nose, and penis. While podiatrists and plastic surgeons use epinephrine in the toes and other parts just mentioned, there is enough controversy about it that I recommend avoiding it. For longer acting anesthesia (3 to 8 hours), however, bupivicaine 0.25% - 0.5% is indicated. All of the blocks that involve the teeth, for example, require long acting anesthesia in order to give your patients pain relief until they can get to the dentist. The maximum dosage of lidocaine with epinephrine for local anesthesia should not exceed 7mg/kg and the maximum total dose should never exceed 500mg. Lidocaine dosage without epinephrine should not exceed 4.5mg/kg and the maximum dose should never exceed 300mg. If the max dosage is ever reached, you can not administer lidocaine again to the same patient for over 2 (two) hours.

A note on topical anesthesia

Use EMLA cream, a topical mixture of lidocaine and prilocaine, only on pediatric patients. Children seem to fear needle punctures more than adults. EMLA cream greatly improves the pediatric nerve blocking experience. I would not suggest extending the use of EMLA to any other patient group as it is relatively expensive and must be applied liberally to the area injected in order to have an adequate anesthetic effect. More importantly, it can take up to 60 minutes to reach its maximum impact. Sixty minutes of waiting time in the Emergency Department does not justify using EMLA cream outside of the pediatric patient population. Should I add bicarbonate to decrease pain? Raising the pH of an anesthetic by adding bicarbonate is known to decrease pain during injection. The correct ratio is 1cc of sodium bicarbonate (1mmol/ml) for every 10cc of lidocaine. When creating this mixture, be sure to wipe the tops of each bottle with alcohol prior to withdrawing the sodium bicarbonate or the lidocaine. Also, prepare to use this mixture immediately. Although some authors suggest that it will keep if refrigerated for up to one week, the risk of growing bacteria and then causing iatrogenic infection does not merit ever saving a buffered anesthetic solution in the refrigerator. Also, do not use sodium bicarbonate with bupivicaine for two reasons. First, it is known to cause a precipitate when combined with bupivicaine rendering the mixture useless. Second, it can decrease the duration of anesthesia which is precisely the opposite goal. In this manual, I suggest using bupivicaine for long acting pain relief in the case of a severe toothache, for example.

Peak effects from anesthesia

Keep in mind that it can take 20 to 30 minutes after performing a peripheral block to achieve the maximum anesthetic effect. I recommend doing the block first then writing up the chart, seeing another patient and then returning to perform the procedure for which the anesthesia was indicated. This will allow enough time for maximum benefits from the anesthetic used.

Why use epinephrine

The use of epinephrine makes the anesthetic effect last longer. Epinephrine causes vasoconstriction which reduces systemic absorption of the anesthetic. Because it vasoconstricts, it also decreases bleeding from the surrounding tissue giving better visualization and a "drier field." Important contraindications to peripheral nerve blocks: patient refusal, infection at site, coagulopathy (relative), allergy to available local anesthetic, existing neurological injury, and lack of knowledge or skill in performing the block.

Nerve block complications and how to prevent them

Nerve injury:

Prevent it by not injecting the anesthetic if your patient reports pain or paresthesia once you insert the needle. Withdraw the needle first, as explained above. Also, don't inject if there is resistance to the anesthetic going in as this indicates high pressure.

Intravascular injection:

Prevent it by aspirating first and withdrawing the needle if blood returns into the syringe.

Hematoma:

Prevent it by using the smallest caliber needle possible. I prefer the 25-ga.

Infection:
Prevent it by always using sterile technique when performing nerve blocks.

Anesthetic toxicity:
Prevent it by never exceeding maximum dosages of anesthetic.

Allergic reaction:
Prevent it by asking your patients if they are allergic to the anesthetic you are about to use.

Other injury:
Prevent it by making sure your patient going home is aware to avoid banging desensate body part against anything and to avoid extreme heat or extreme cold contact. Always make sure that the body part having received anesthesia has adequate padding and is positioned or splinted to prevent inadvertent injury.

Before performing a nerve block

Prior to injecting a patient always perform a complete neurological exam and document any sensory or motor deficits. Always inform the patient that any sensory or motor dysfunction you identify during physical exam may be permanent. Make sure to document your neurological exam in the permanent medical record. Remember that an existing neurological injury is a contraindication to performing a nerve block.

Patient consent

For local, peripheral anesthesia in the emergency department or urgent care, verbal consent is sufficient. Consent obtained verbally, however, should be documented. Even if the block is done for pain management alone, verbal consent should be obtained and charted. You should write that the patient was advised about the risk of local anesthetic toxicity (rash or other form of allergic reaction), and that possible nerve injury from the block itself was explained.

A separate note for peripheral nerve blocks

I suggest writing a separate note for the peripheral nerve block itself. This note should include the specific nerve that was blocked and the reason the block was performed. You must also be explicit about the type of needle used (25-ga), the type and the amount of local anesthesia injected.

The "Patient Consent," just described, should be documented in this note. When a separate note is included in this manner, it communicates you considered the case more carefully and performed an additional procedure in order to manage pain properly. This can translate into a separate reimbursement that you otherwise would not receive if you had chosen local infiltration.

HAND BLOCKS

SENSATION OF THE HAND

FIG 1A

FIG 1B

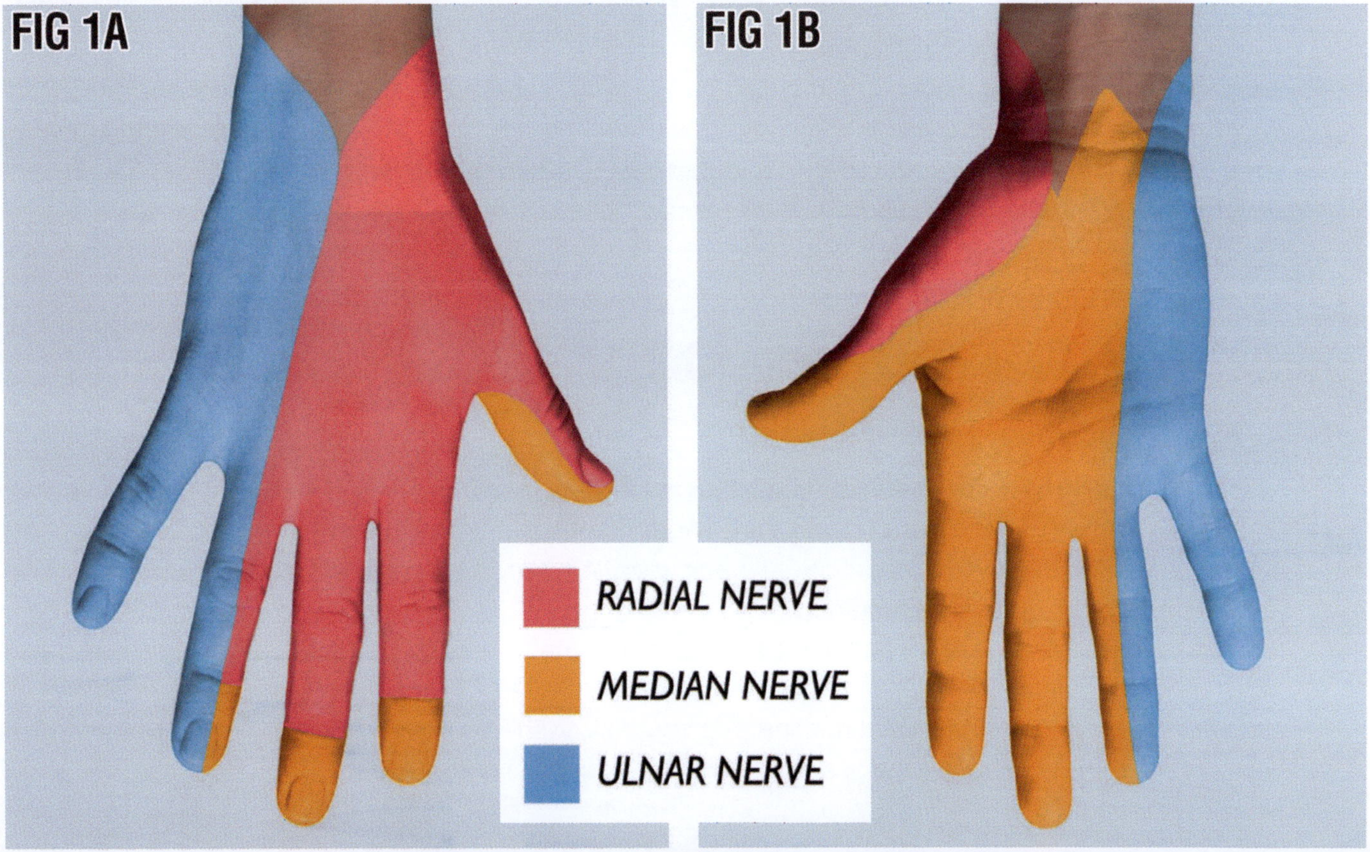

Sensory Distribution of Radial Nerve:

Blocking the radial nerve at the level of the wrist will provide anesthesia to the dorsum of the hand from the thumb up to one half of the fourth digit. Sensation beyond the distal interphalangeal joints (DIP) of the three middle fingers is not covered by the radial nerve, and therefore will not be blocked. On the volar aspect of the hand, the radial nerve does cover a sliver of the thenar eminence.
See FIG 1A and FIG 1B.

Radial Nerve Block (Volar Approach):

- Insert a 25-ga needle just lateral to the palpable radial artery at the level of the proximal wrist crease (PWC). Your point of entry should be perpendicular to the wrist.
- Maintain your non-dominant index and third finger tips on the radial pulse. At the depth of the artery, inject 5cc of anesthetic (FIG 2). Then pull back without removing the needle from the skin and inject another 5 cc of anesthetic SQ, pointing and advancing the needle towards the dorsum of the wrist.
- Stay at the level of the PWC. Remove the needle from the initial point of entry and re-enter at a point more dorsal, again staying at the level of the PWC.
- Advance the needle to the dorsal midline of the wrist and then withdraw to this second point of entry while injecting an additional 3cc of anesthetic. The goal here is to create a field block from the initial point of entry to the dorsal midline of the wrist (FIG 3).

RADIAL NERVE BLOCK

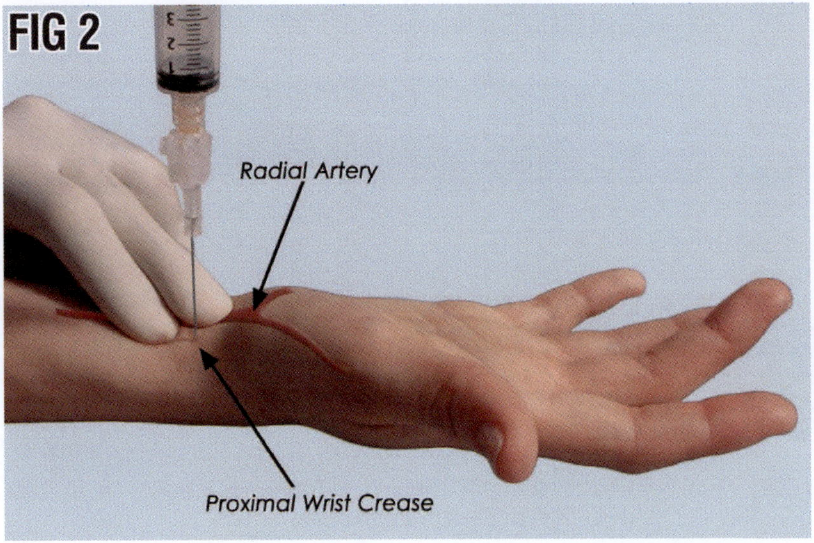

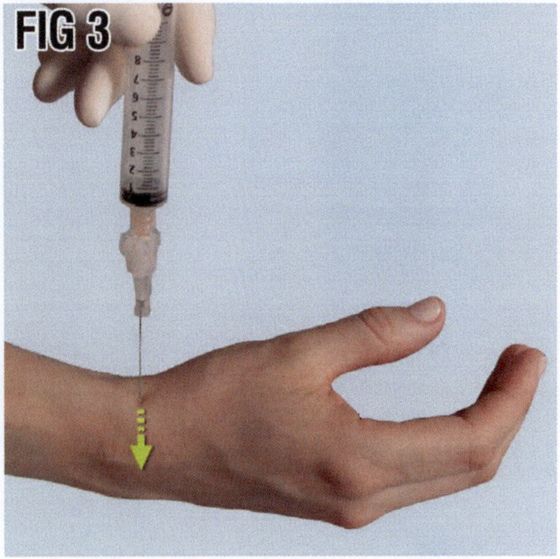

Sensory Distribution of Ulnar Nerve:

Blocking the ulnar nerve at the level of the wrist will provide anesthesia to the dorsal and ventral hand from the fifth digit to one-half of the fourth digit. See FIG 1A and FIG 1B.

Ulnar Nerve Block (Lateral Approach):

- First locate the flexor carpi ulnaris tendon by having your patient flex the wrist against resistance. The tendon can be easily palpated on the ulnar aspect of the wrist right under the pisiform bone.
- Insert a 25-ga needle on the ulnar aspect and under the flexor carpi ulnaris for a distance of 1.0 cm. Go in at the level of the proximal wrist crease (PWC) and aim the needle towards the ulnar bone.
- At this point inject 3cc to 5cc of anesthetic. (FIG 4) Keep in mind that the ulnar nerve runs along the radial aspect of the flexor carpi ulnaris. You must get under the tendon and the tip of the needle must reach the location of the nerve in order for the block to be successful.
- After depositing anesthetic, pull back the needle without removing it from the skin and advance it towards the dorsal midline of the wrist, always remaining at the level of the PWC.
- Withdraw the needle to its initial point of entry, depositing an additional 5cc of anesthetic. The goal with this second injection is to cover a field from the the dorsal midline of the wrist to the lateral border of the flexor carpi ulnaris tendon (FIG 5).

ULNAR NERVE BLOCK

FIG 4

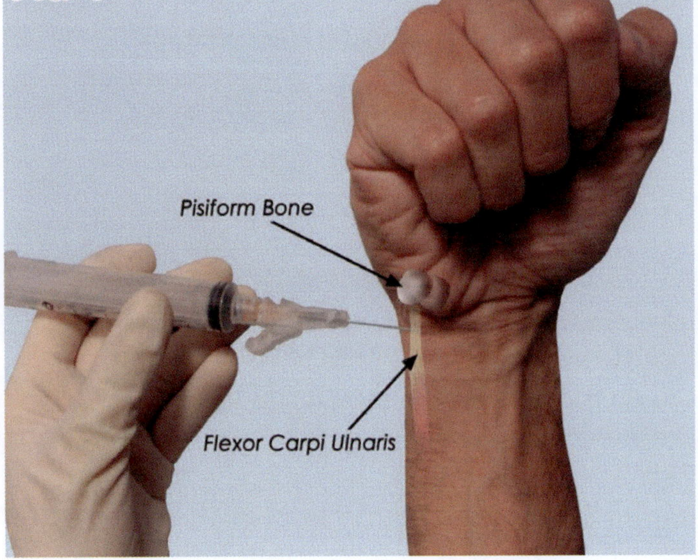

FIG 5

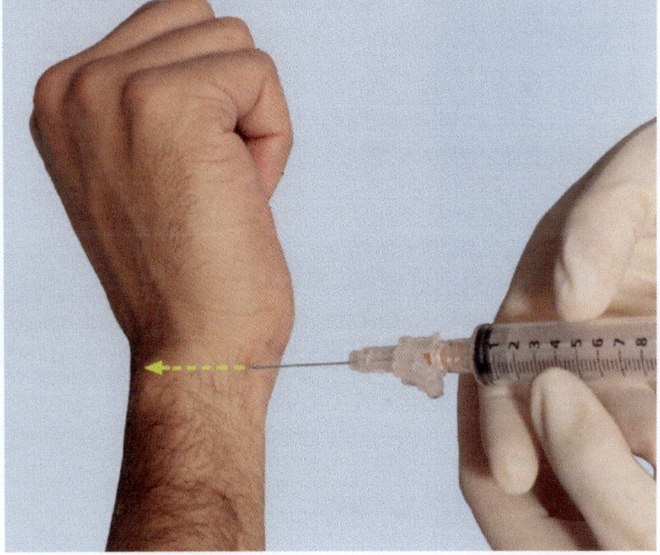

Sensory Distribution of Median Nerve:

Blocking the median nerve at the level of the wrist provides anesthesia to the dorsal three middle digits beyond the DIP joint and the ventral hand from the thumb to one-half of the fourth digit. Sensation to a small portion of the thenar eminence is not covered by the median nerve.
See FIG 1A and FIG 1B.

Median Nerve Block:

- Locate the flexor palmaris longus and the flexor carpi radialis tendons. The ”radialis” reminds you that this tendon is the one more radial than the other. Both of these can be found by having your patient flex the wrist during palpation. The palmaris longus tendon will protrude more if you have your patient oppose the thumb to the tip of the fifth digit.
- Insert the needle between the two tendons 0.5cm proximal to the proximal wrist crease and stay perpendicular to the wrist. Aim posteriorly towards the deep fascia. Be sure to feel for a ”pop” to make sure that you have penetrated the retinaculum. Inject 3cc to 5cc of anesthetic at this point.

Note: Twenty percent (20%) of your patients will not have a flexor palmaris longus. In these cases your point of entry is 1cm ulnar from the ulnar edge of the flexor carpi radialis at the same level just described (FIG 6).

MEDIAN NERVE BLOCK

FIG 6

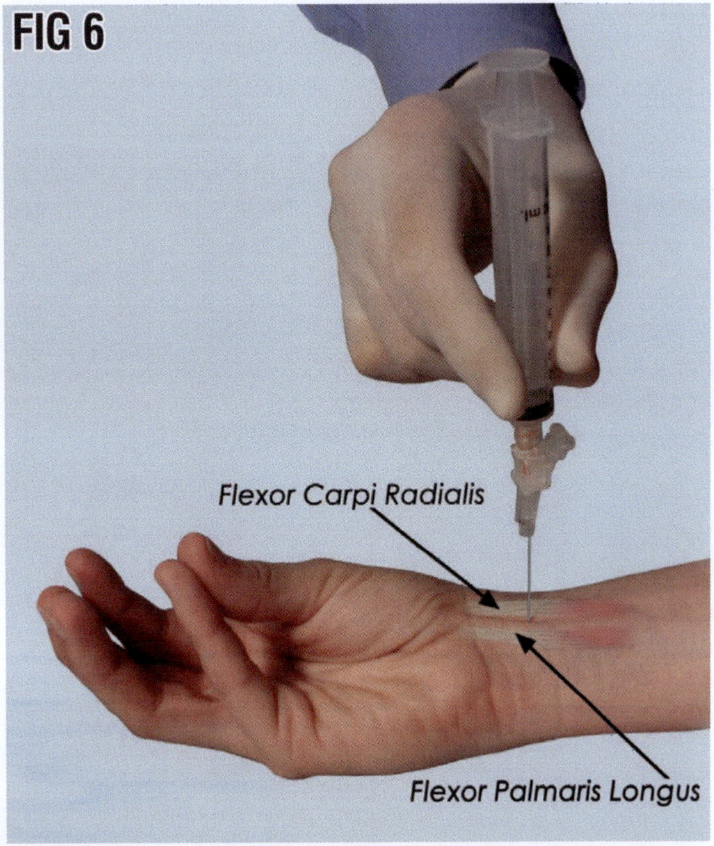

Digital Nerve Blocks:

- Insert a 25-ga needle directly over the palmar, metacarpal head, and position the needle centrally. Your point of entry should be at the distal aspect of the metacarpal head and remain perpendicular to the palm. Inject anesthesia as needle approaches the bone.
- Pull back needle about 4 mm and direct needle to the left and then to the right, injecting more anesthesia on either side.
- Use about 5cc total to block one digit. This approach can be used for anyone of the three middle fingers, except it will leave the most proximal, dorsal surfaces with some sensation.
- In order to properly block the thumb and fifth digit, start with the same palmar approach just described above for the three middle digits (FIG 7). Then, for the thumb or fifth digit, insert the needle into the corresponding dorsal web space just beyond the knuckle.
- Inject 1cc of anesthetic adjacent to the first or fifth digit respectively in this web space. (FIG 8) Then pull back a few millimeters and move the needle and advance it over the top of phalanx injecting 1cc adjacent to the radial edge of the first digit or the ulnar edge of the fifth digit (FIG 9). Stay just distal to the knuckles throughout this approach. If full anesthesia of the most proximal, dorsal three middle fingers is desired you must implement the dorsal injection just described for the thumb and fifth digit to the three middle digits. Keep in mind that in most cases I am able to get proper anesthesia of the three middle fingers using the palmar approach by itself. In the hand, I always massage the injected area to improve diffusion of anesthetic throughout the tissues.

DIGITAL NERVE BLOCK

FIG 7

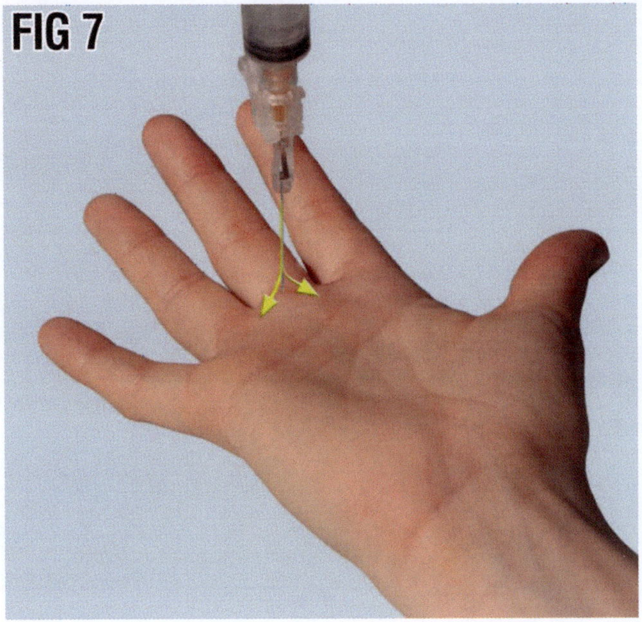

FIG 8

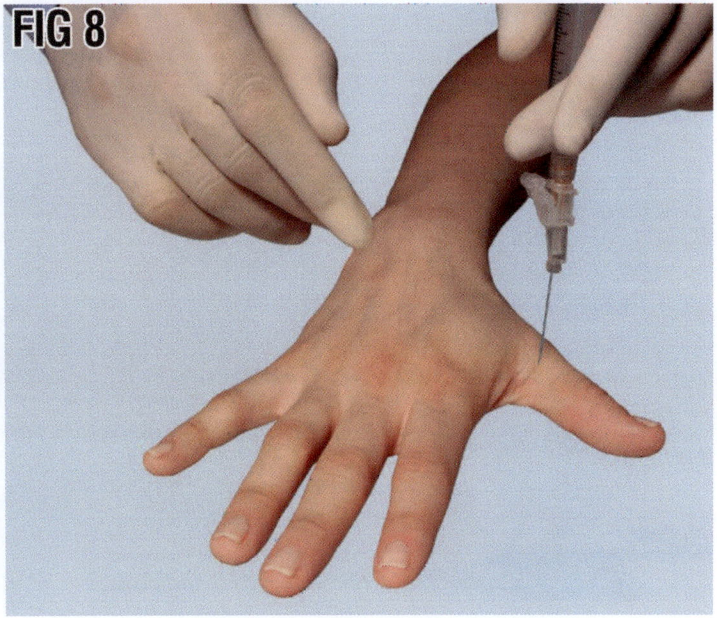

DIGITAL NERVE BLOCK (continued)

FIG 9

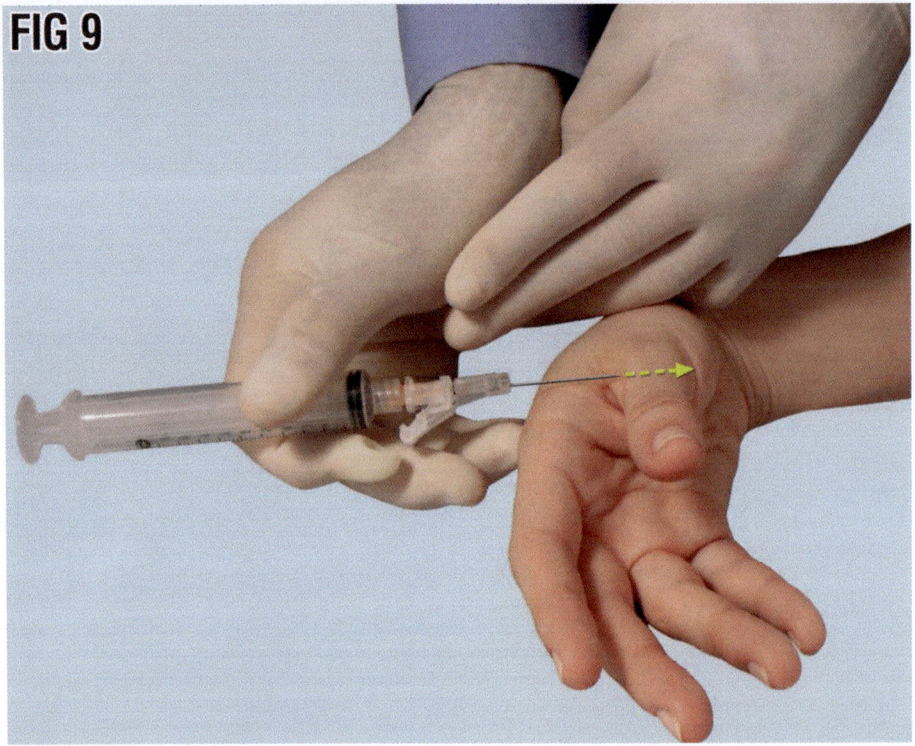

CUTANEOS SENSATION OF THE FOOT

Sural Nerve
Posterior Tibial Nerve
Saphenous Nerve
Anterior Tibial Nerve
Superficial Peroneal Nerve

Sensory Distribution of Sural Nerve:

Blocking the sural nerve will provide anesthesia to the heel and the posterior lateral aspect of the foot and ankle (FIG 10).

Sural Nerve Block:

- Insert a 25-ga needle 1cm above the lateral malleolus advancing the needle posteriorly towards the lateral edge of the Achilles tendon.
- Remain subcutaneous. Withdraw the needle to the point of entry while injecting 5cc of anesthetic. The idea is to create a band-like distribution of anesthetic between the Achilles tendon and the lateral malleolus (FIG 11).

SURAL NERVE BLOCK

FIG 10

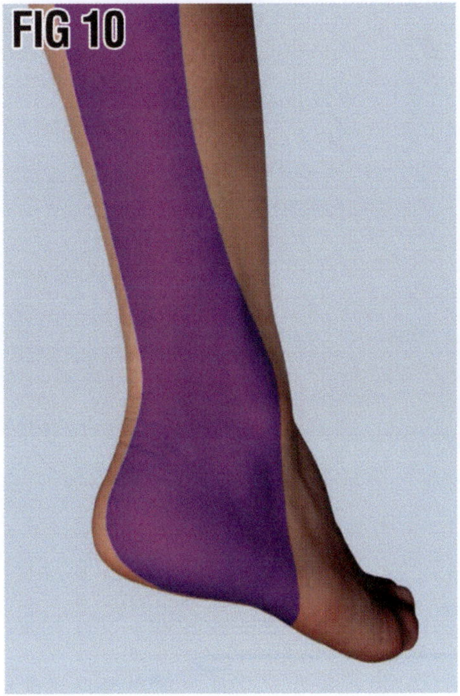

FIG 11

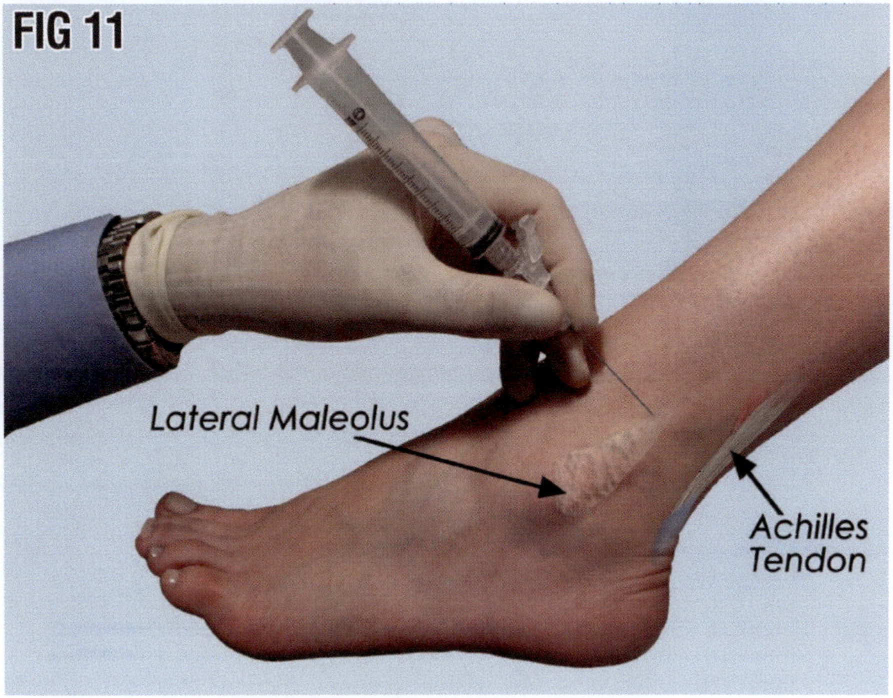

Sensory Distribution of Posterior Tibial Nerve:

Blocking the posterior tibial nerve will provide anesthesia to almost the entire sole of the foot including the distal volar foot and the volar skin of all the toes. It does not provide anesthesia to the heel or the extreme medial or the extreme lateral aspects of the sole (FIG 12).

Posterior Tibial Nerve Block:

- Place the patient prone to carry out this procedure.
- Insert a 25-ga needle (at least 3cm long) between the medial border of the Achilles tendon and the posterior tibial artery (PTA). Stay at the level of the superior aspect of the medial malleolus.
- Position your hand holding the syringe just posterior to the heel and insert at the medial edge of the Achilles tendon advancing anteriorly. Keep the needle just adjacent to the posterior edge of the PTA without cannulating it.
- Advance the needle to the tibia. Once the needle comes into contact with the tibia, withdraw about 1mm and aspirate to make sure you are not in the PTA.
- Then inject 7cc at this location as you withdraw the needle for 1cm (FIG 13).

POSTERIOR TIBIAL NERVE BLOCK

FIG 12

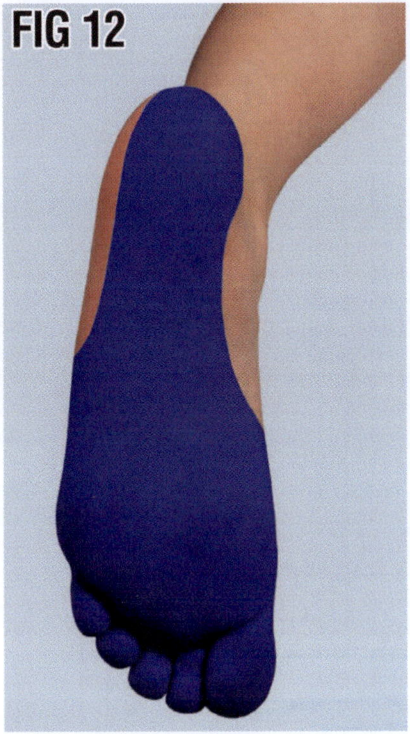

FIG 13

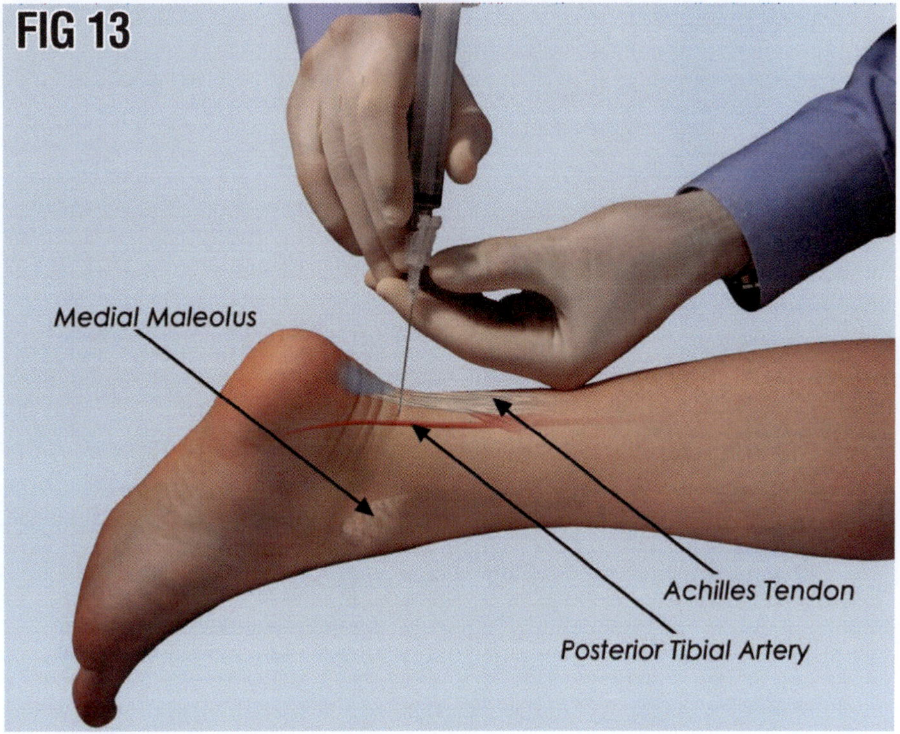

Sensory Distribution of Saphenous Nerve:

Blocking the saphenous nerve will provide anesthesia to the medial aspect of the foot, including the arch (FIG 14).

Saphenous Nerve Block:

Note: Before attempting this block, find your own anterior tibialis tendon to gain confidence that you are precise about your landmarks.

- In a seated position bend over and place the fingertips of your dominant hand on the anterior corresponding ankle.
- Evert the foot and palpate the protruding anterior tibialis tendon. Note that this tendon is a bit more medial than one would otherwise expect (FIG 15). Instructions continue on page 32.

SAPHENOUS NERVE BLOCK

FIG 14

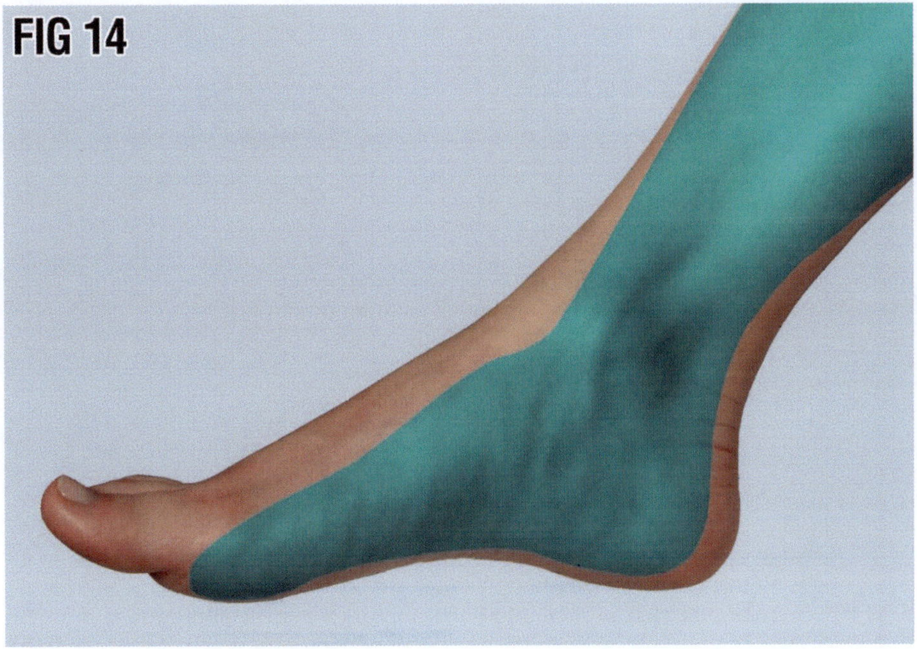

FIG 15

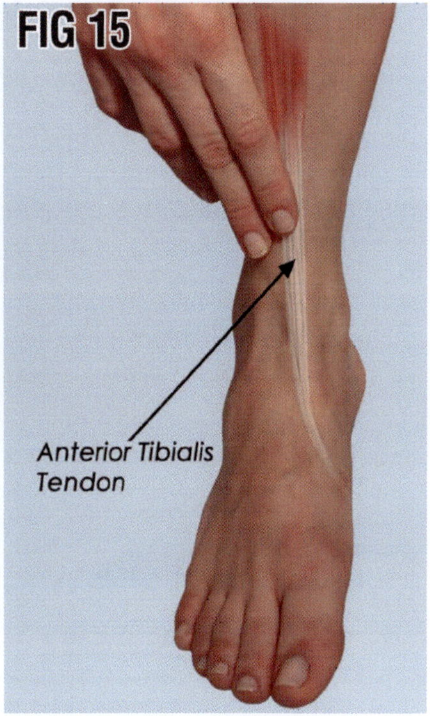

Saphenous Nerve Block:

- Insert a 25-ga needle (at least 3cm long) at a level 1cm superior to the medial malleolus. Your point of entry should be the medial edge of the anterior tibialis tendon.
- Advance the needle posteriorly and towards the tibia so that the needle contacts the bone at a point midline between the medial edge of the anterior tibialis tendon and 1cm above the medial malleolus.
- Once the needle comes in contact with the tibia withdraw 2mm and inject 2cc of anesthetic at this location. Then inject an additional 5cc total in a band-like pattern, subcutaneously, between the anterior tibialis tendon and the medial maleolus, the whole time remain 1cm superior to the medial malleolus (FIG 16).

SAPHENOUS NERVE BLOCK

FIG 16

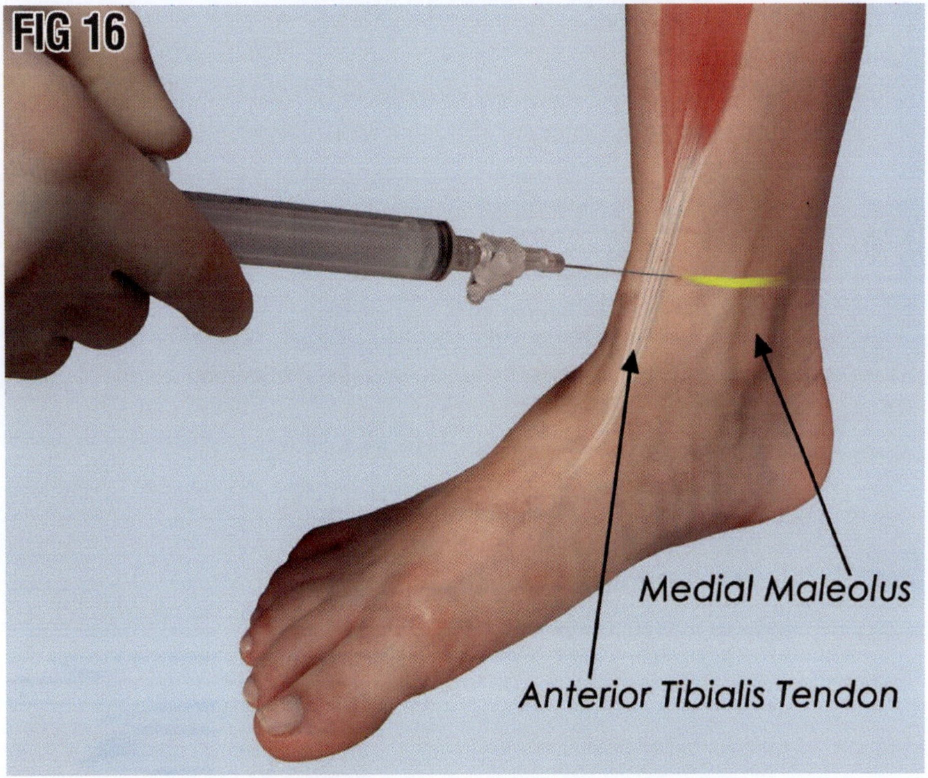

Sensory Distribution of Anterior Tibial Nerve:

Blocking the Anterior Tibial Nerve will provide anesthesia to the dorsal web space between the first and second toes (FIG 17).

Anterior Tibial Nerve Block:

- Position your hand holding the syringe in front of the ankle. Insert a 25-ga needle immediately lateral to the anterior tibialis tendon, 1cm superior to the medial malleolus.
- Direct the needle laterally until you reach the tibia.
- Withdraw the needle 1mm and inject 4cc of anesthetic at this location (FIG 18).

ANTERIOR TIBIAL NERVE BLOCK

FIG 17

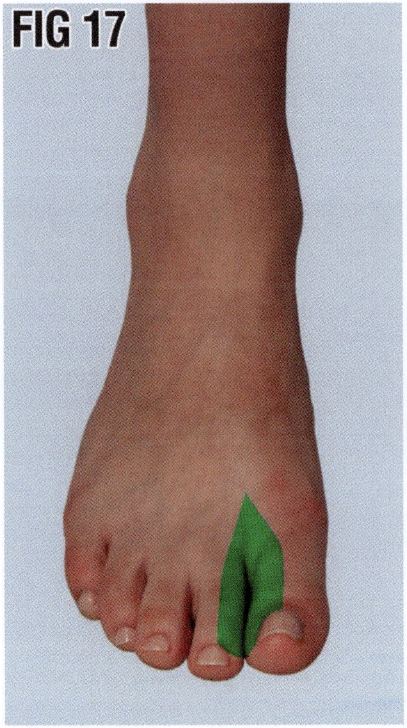

FIG 18

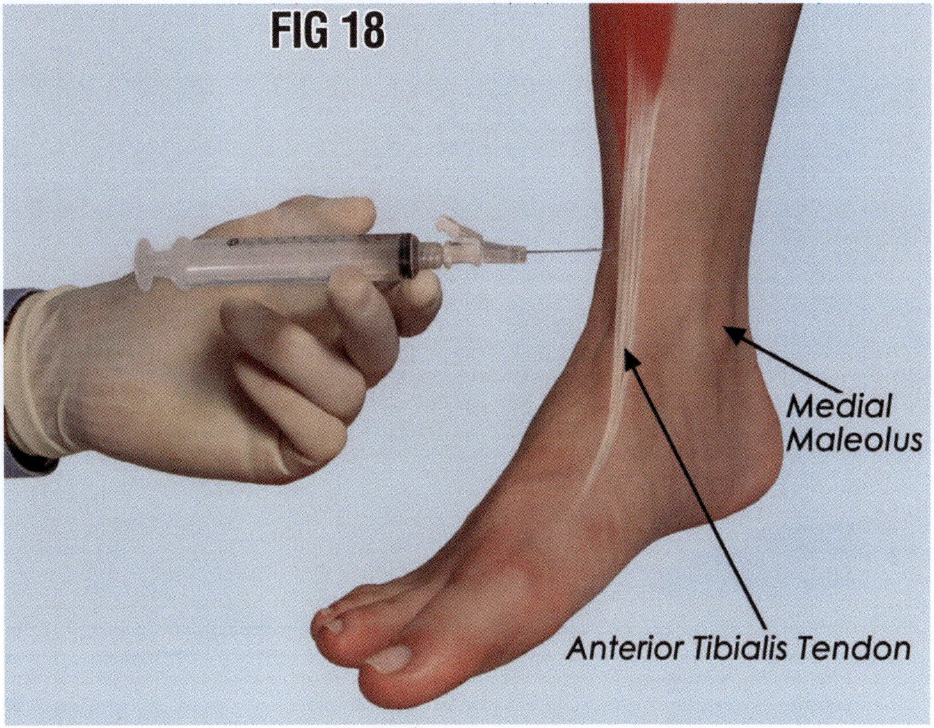

Sensory Distribution of Superficial Peroneal Nerve:

Blocking the superficial peroneal nerve will provide anesthesia to the dorsal foot, excluding the dorsal web space between the first and second toes (FIG 19).

Superficial Peroneal Nerve Block:

- Insert a 25-ga needle at the level of the ankle perpendicular to the long axis of the foot. Your point of entry is just lateral to the extensor hallucis longus tendon.
- Advance the needle towards the lateral malleolus and remain subcutaneous the whole time.
- Inject 10cc of anesthetic as you withdraw the needle in order to provide anesthetic in a band-like distribution between these two landmarks (FIG 20).

SUPERFICIAL PERONEAL NERVE BLOCK

FIG 19

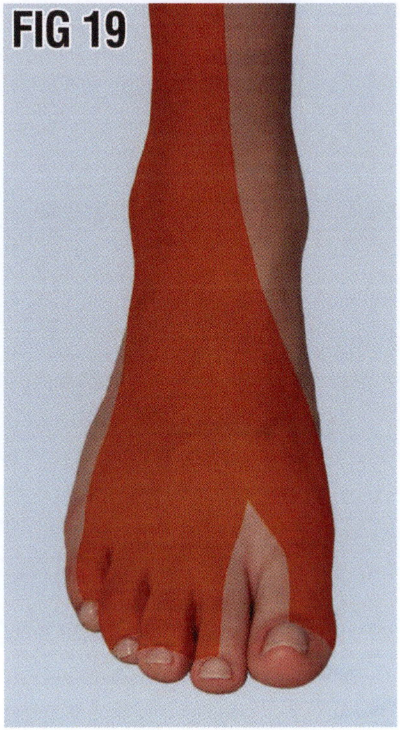

FIG 20

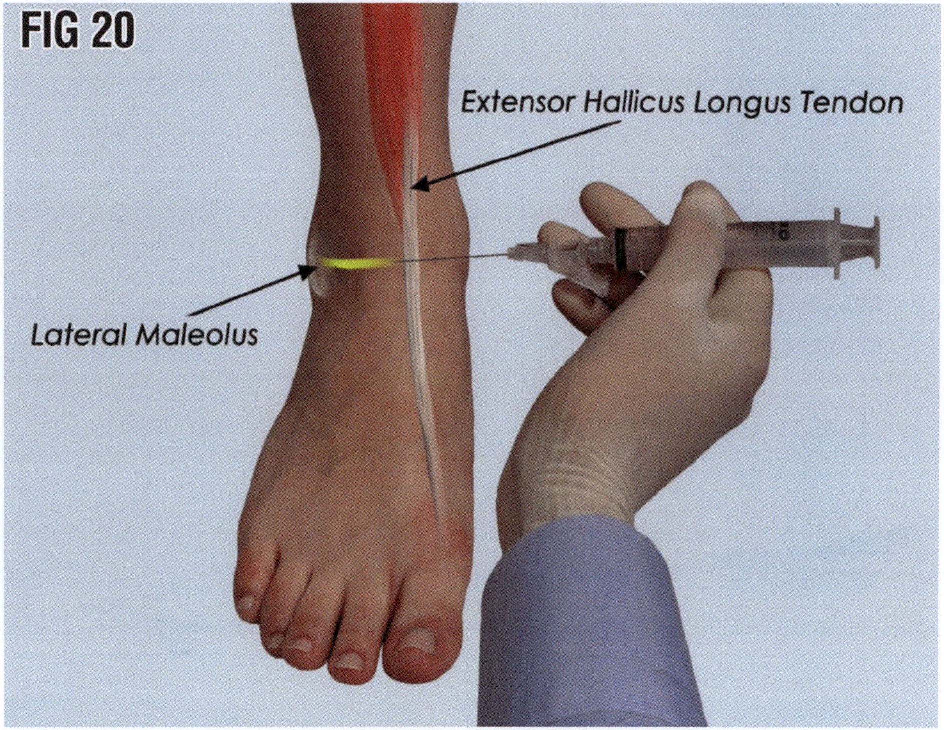

Nerve Blocks of the Toes:

- Use the digital web spaces. Insert a 25-ga needle on both sides of the toe requiring anesthesia.
- Position the needle at the most distal edge of the metatarsals or the most proximal edge of the web spaces and on the dorsal side of the foot.
- Start with 1cc of anesthetic close to the dorsal surface and then advance the needle until there is some tenting of the volar skin. Then inject an additional 2cc as the needle is withdrawn.
- Re-advance the needle at a different angle towards the volar skin within the same web space and inject additional anesthetic as you withdraw the needle (FIG 21). The idea is to inject in a fan-like distribution for each web-space receiving anesthesia.
  (SEE CROSS-SECTION)

For the first and fifth toes, anesthesia using the same technique just described must be carried out on the lateral aspects of each metatarsal respectively. Even on the lateral sides of the first and fifth metatarsals the needle must be withdrawn and re-advanced at a new angle with the point tilted towards the midline of the sole. Deposit more anesthetic each time you re-advance the needle at a different angle.

TOE NERVE BLOCK

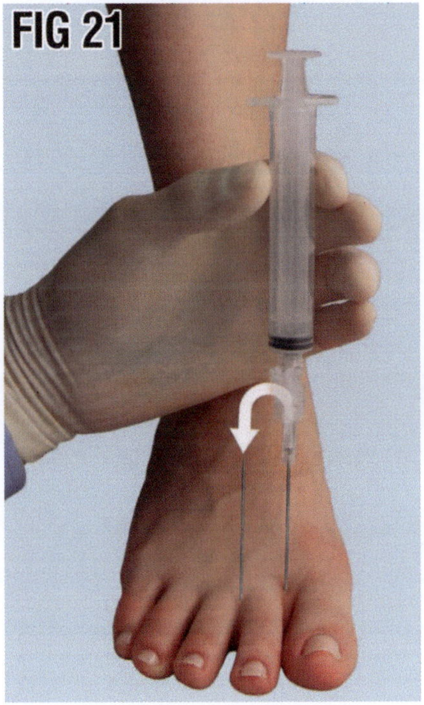

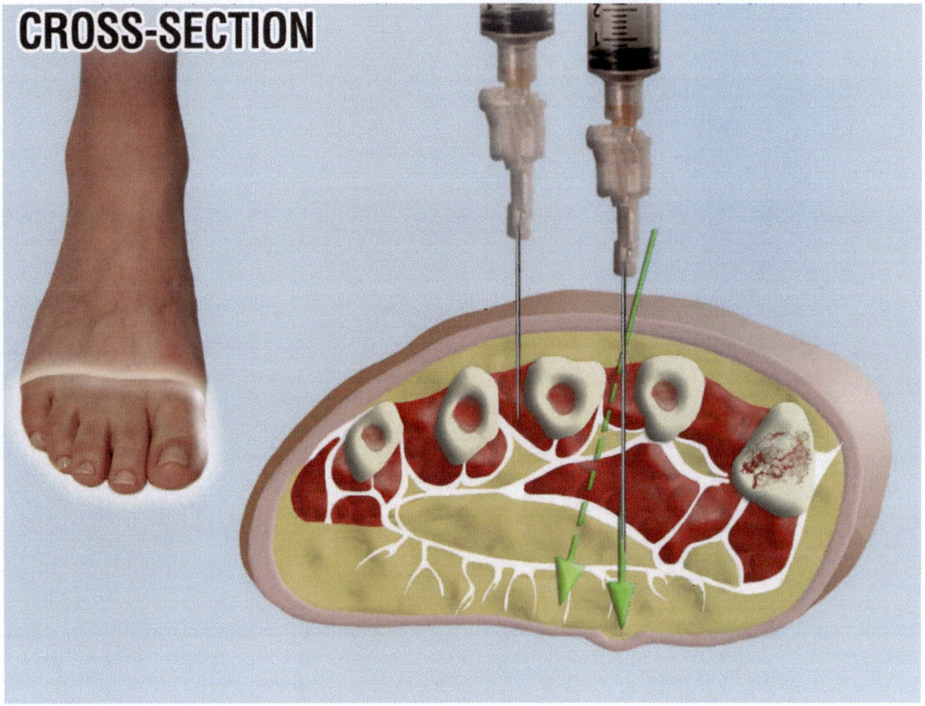

FACIAL BLOCKS

Sensory Distribution of Supraorbital Nerve:

Blocking the supraorbital nerve at the supraorbital notch provides anesthesia to the forehead, anterior scalp, medial canthus, lateral nose, nasal root, and upper eyelid for each respective side (FIG 22).

Supraorbital Nerve Block:

- First find the supraorbital notch by palpating along the medial aspect of the supraorbital rim.
- Keep in mind that's where the nerve exists and branches cephalad to cover the territory requiring anesthesia.
- Insert a 27-ga or 25-ga needle at the medial edge of the lateral third of the eyebrow.
- Keep the needle at a 15 degree angle from the forehead and advance it medially to the medial canthus. The whole time remain horizontal over the eyebrow.
- Inject 2cc of anesthetic at this location (FIG 23).

SUPRAORBITAL NERVE BLOCK

FIG 22

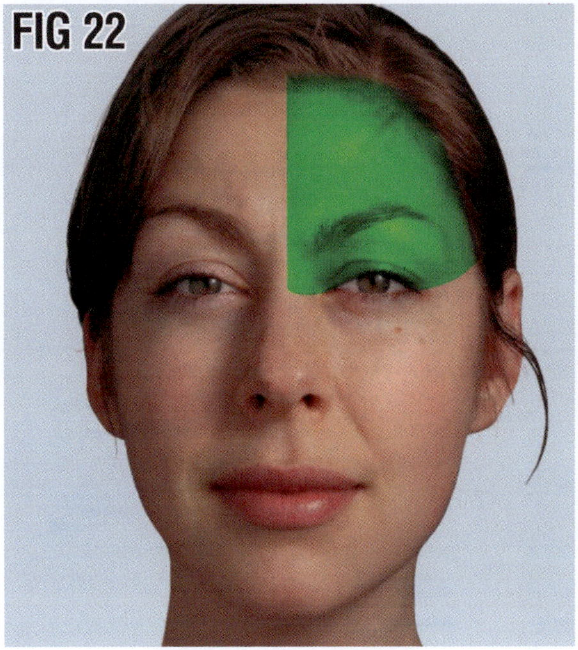

FIG 23

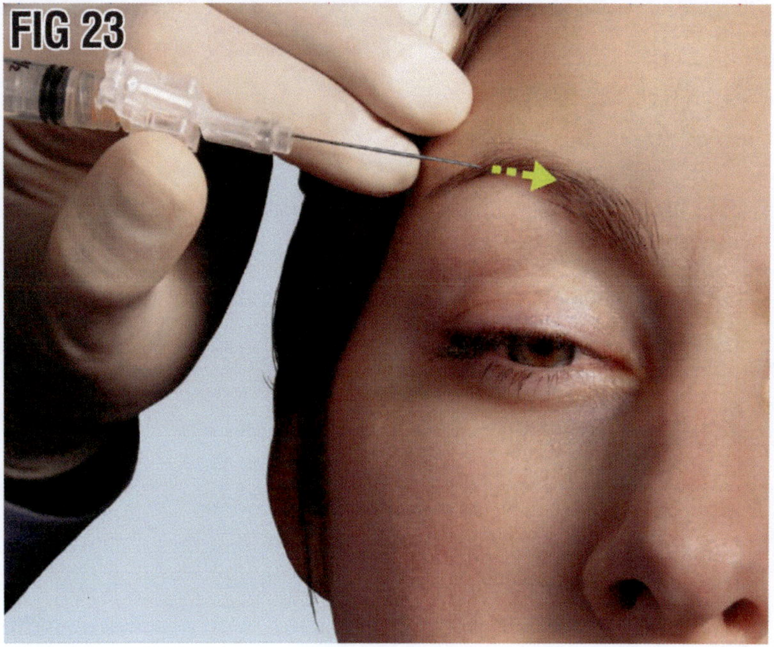

Sensory Distribution of Infraorbital Nerve:

Blocking the inferior orbital nerve will provide anesthesia to the lateral nose, the upper lip, medial cheek, lower eyelid, and upper teeth for each respective side (FIG 25).

Infraorbital Nerve Block:

I prefer the intraoral approach rather than transcutaneous.

- Place the third fingertip of the non-dominant hand on the infraorbital foramen.
- Lift the lip with the index finger and thumb.
- Position the needle over the second bicuspid tooth and insert at the gingival buccal sulcus.
- Advance the needle superiorly towards the third fingertip marking the foramen and inject 2cc of anesthetic.
- The whole time remain in line with the vertical axis of the tooth (FIG 26).

INFRAORBITAL NERVE BLOCK

FIG 25

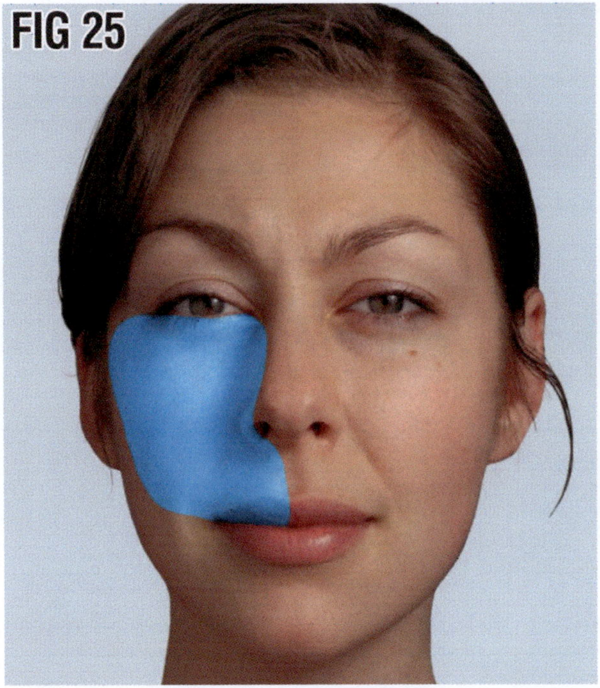

FIG 26

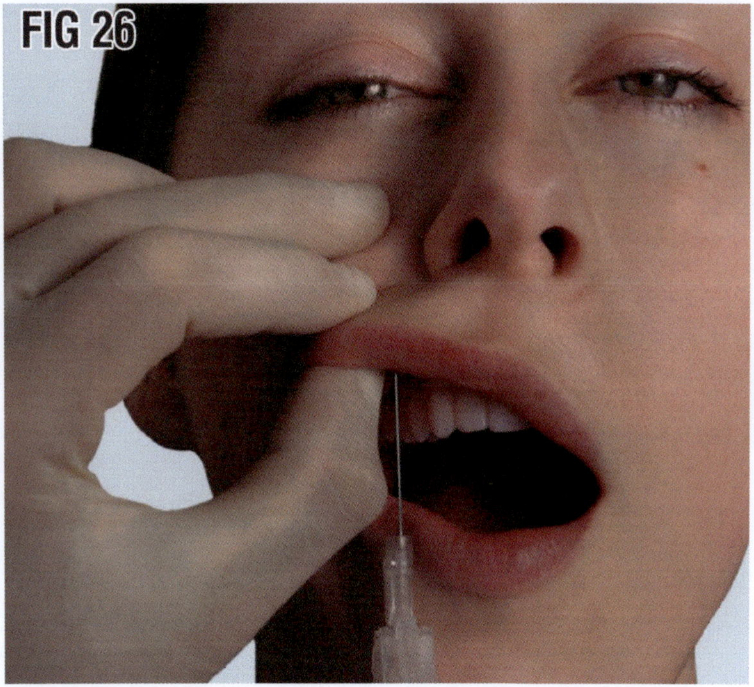

Sensory Distribution of the Nose:

Blocking the nerves that supply the nose with sensation can be accomplished with two injections that are relatively less painful than attempting to inject anesthetic anywhere near the tip of the nose. This block provides anesthesia to the entire nose distal to the nasal bone (FIG 27).

Nasal Block:

- Using the thumb and index finger of the non-dominant hand pinch the nose, palpating for the nasal bone at the point where it meets the most proximal edge of the nasal cartilage.
- Insert a 25-ga needle at this level, 8mm from the midline, then inject 2cc of anesthetic.
- Withdraw the needle and repeat this technique on the other side of the nose, 8mm from the midline and inject an additional 2cc of anesthetic (FIG 28).

NASAL NERVE BLOCK

FIG 27

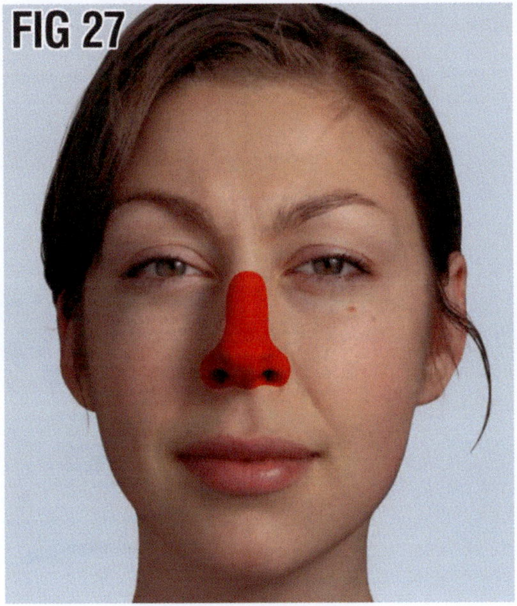

FIG 28

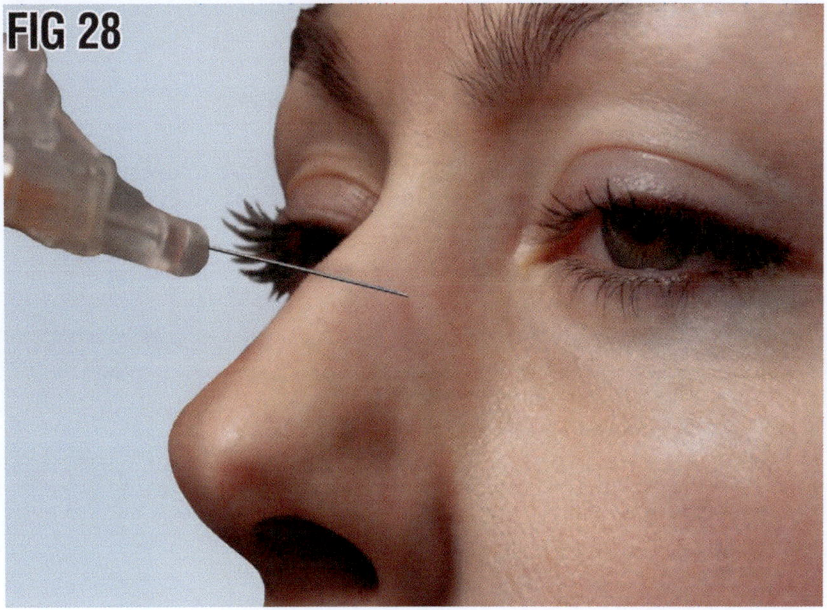

Sensory Distribution of the Mental Nerve:

Blocking the mental nerve will provide anesthesia to the lower lip and chin for each respective side (FIG 30).

Mental Nerve Block:

- For the mental nerve, I prefer the intraoral approach.
- Make sure your patient's mouth is open.
- Using the index finger and thumb of the non-dominant hand grab the lower lip and pull it anteriorly.
- Insert a 25-ga needle 5mm inferior to the second bicuspid and inject 2cc of anesthetic at this point. The whole time remain 45 degrees to the vertical axis of the tooth (FIG 31).

MENTAL NERVE BLOCK

FIG 30

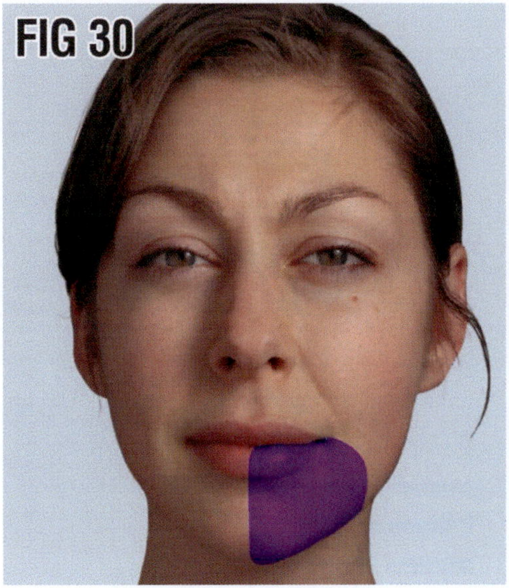

FIG 31

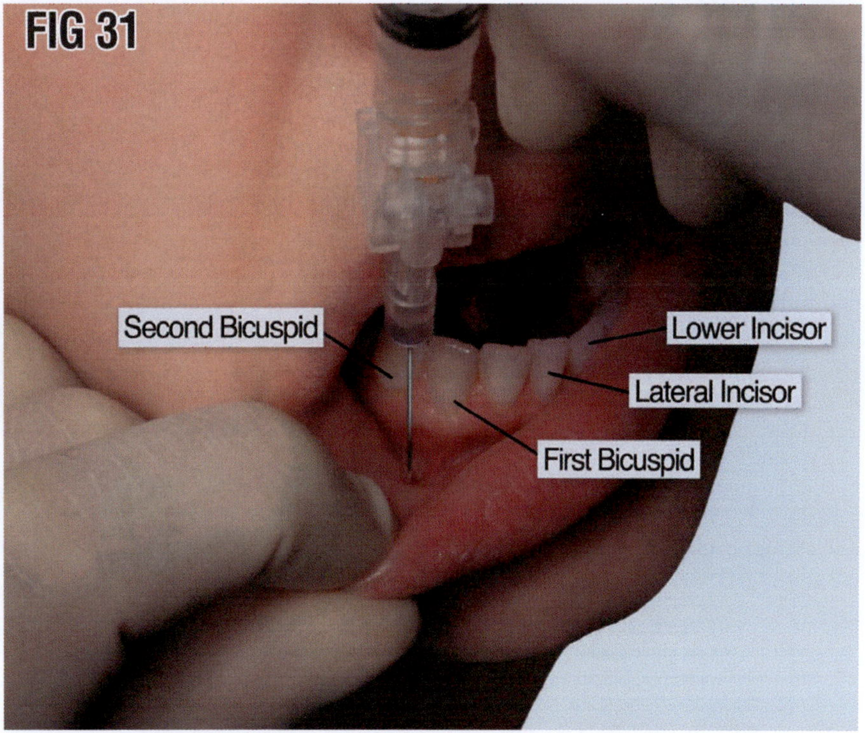

Nerve Block for the Entire Ear:

- Insert a 25-ga needle just inferior to the spot where the earlobe attaches to the head.
- Direct the needle anteriorly towards the tragus and inject 1cc of anesthetic.
- Withdraw the needle without pulling it out of the skin entirely and redirect it along the inferior posterior auricular sulcus, injecting an additional 1cc of anesthetic.
- Then remove the needle and insert at the most superior spot where the auricle attaches to the head. Direct the needle towards tragus and inject 1cc of anesthetic.
- Withdraw the needle without pulling it out of the skin entirely and redirect it along the helix posteriorly, and inject 1cc of anesthetic.
- Never inject the cartilage of the ear itself. Stay clear of the superficial temporal artery located medial to the ear (FIG 32).

Nerve Block of Tragus and Helix only:

- Insert a 25-ga needle just anterior to the tragus and advance it 3mm superiorly towards the helix.
- Remain at a 15 degree angle from the face.
- Inject 2cc of anesthetic (FIG 33).

EAR NERVE BLOCKS

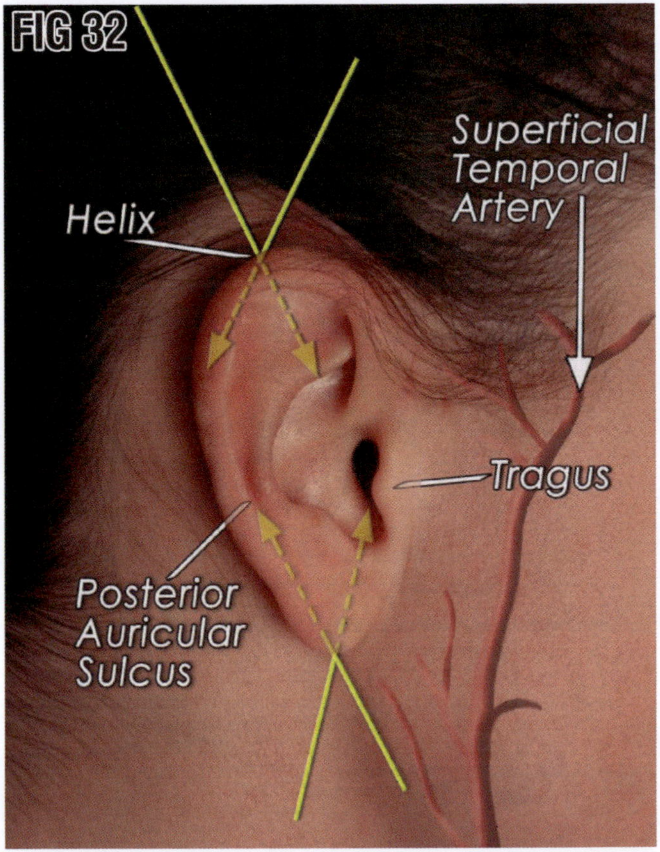

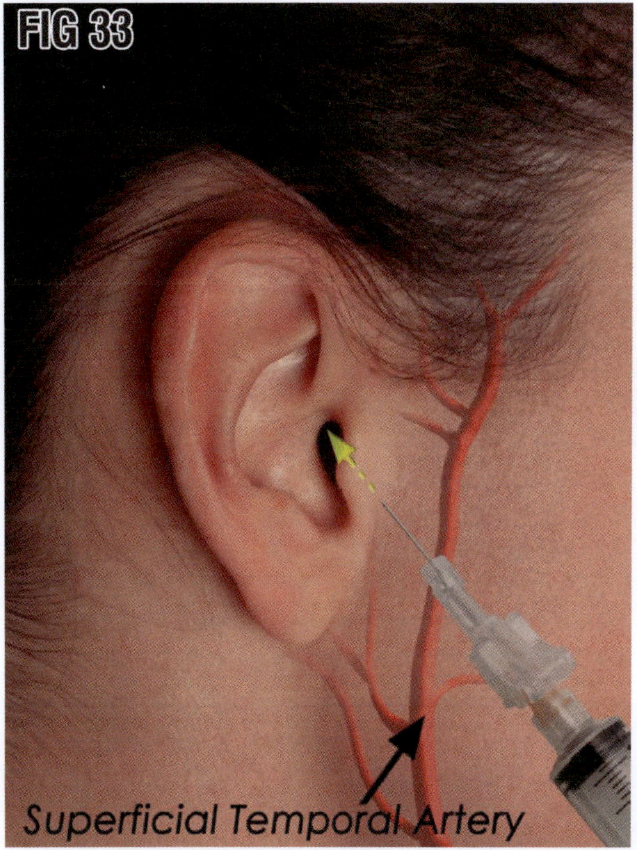

DENTAL BLOCKS

FIG 34

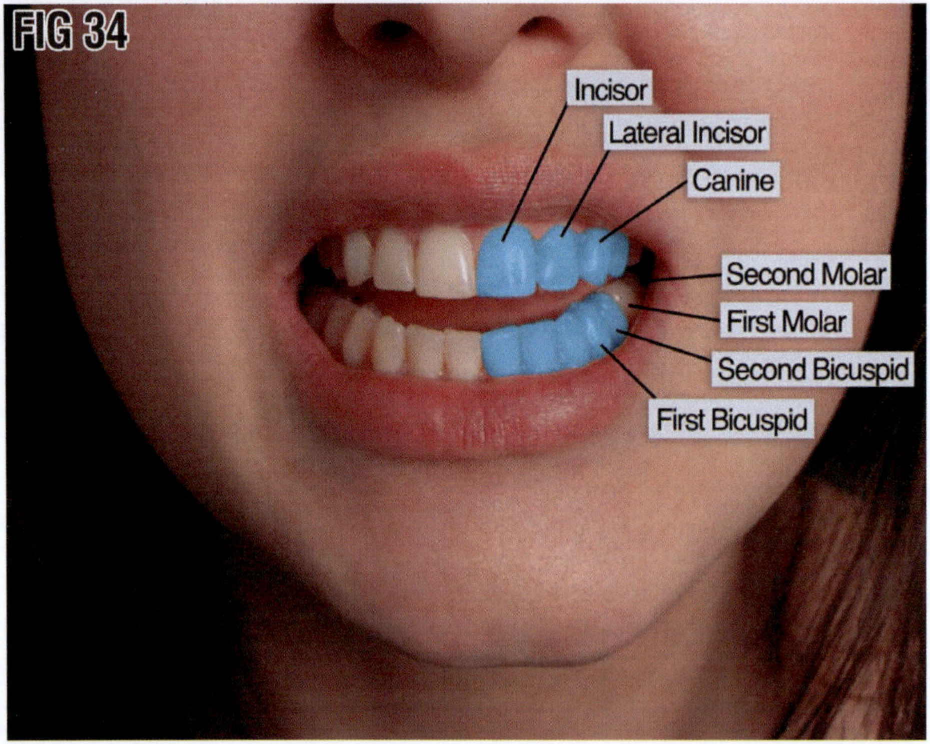

Position of Patient for all Dental Blocks:

In the emergency department or urgent care center where a dental chair is normally not available, place the patient in a seated position and rest the occiput on a raised stretcher or exam table.

Sensory Distribution of Dental and Gingivial Nerve Branches:

Blocking dental and gingival nerve branches will provide anesthesia to the maxillary or mandibular teeth: incisors, canines, and bicuspids.

Why block sensory nerves of the teeth:

In emergency medicine, tooth pain either from fracture, periapical or periodontal infection is so common I feel it is essential that all ED physicians are able and willing to offer their patients a long acting 0.5% Bupivicaine block until they can get to a dentist.

We tend to give these patients two percocets in the ER and percocets to go. The block, in my opinion, is a cleaner more effective approach for pain relief.

Dental / Gingival Nerve Branch Block (for maxillary / mandibular incisors, canines, and bicuspids):

- Insert a 25-ga needle immediately posterior to the affected tooth at a level that is supraperiosteal, above the tooth in the maxilla and below the tooth in the mandible.
- Pull the lip away and insert the needle into the buccal vestibule and direct it 4mm in towards the root apex.
- Once you have reached the bone withdraw the needle for 1mm and inject 2cc of 0.5% bupivacaine (FIG 35). Wait 20 minutes.
- If the patient continues to report pain, inject supraperiosteal an additional 2cc of anesthetic on the palatal side (FIG 36).

DENTAL/GINGIVIAL NERVE BLOCK

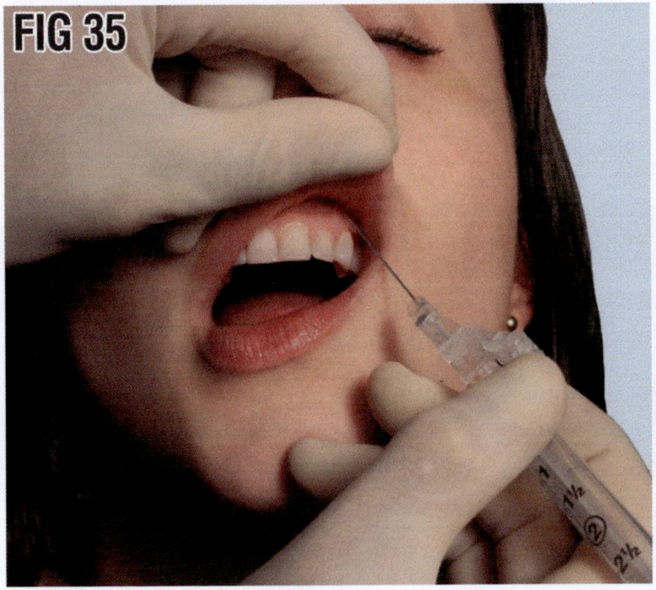

FIG 35

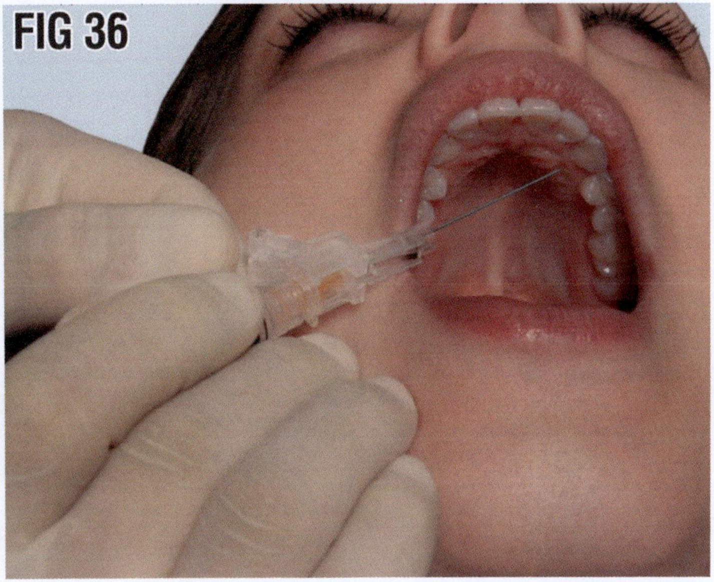
FIG 36

Peridontal Ligament Block (additional anesthesia for maxillary/ mandibular incisors, canines, and bicuspids):

- Use this technique to provide additional anesthesia, if needed, after buccal vestibule and palatal supraperiosteal injections described above.
- Wait an additional 20 minutes to see if additional anesthesia is required (i.e. if your patient is still complaining of pain).
- Pull the lip away and insert needle at the edge of the gingiva and just posterior to the tooth requiring anesthesia.
- Keep the needle as parallel to the tooth as possible.
- Advance the needle superiorly for 1mm to 2mm and inject 0.2cc of anesthetic.
- This injection should be carried out slowly over 25 seconds and expect some resistance (FIG 37).

PERIODONTAL LIGAMENT BLOCK

FIG 37

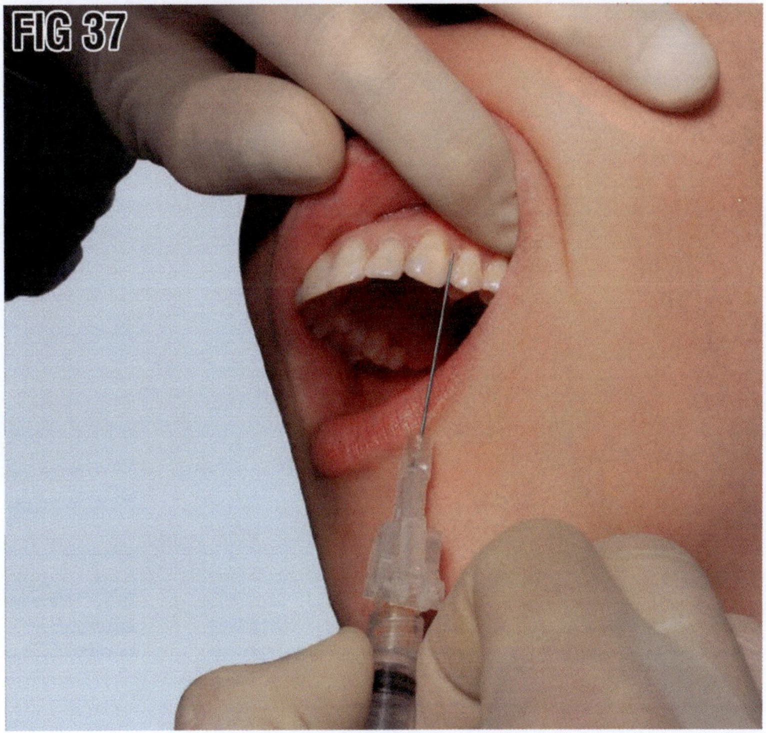

Sensory Distribution of Posterior Superior Alveolar Nerve:

Blocking the posterior superior alveolar nerve provides anesthesia to the molars, except for the most anterior part of the first molar. With enough lip retraction the supraperiosteal approach described earlier (dental/gingival nerve branch block) should be used for the anterior first molar.

If there is inflammation or infection of the maxillary molars, the posterior superior alveolar nerve block is ideal because the point of entry is the posterior oral cavity away from the area where the pain or infection is located.

Posterior Superior Alveolar Nerve Block:

- Retract the lip for the respective side requiring anesthesia.
- Expose the mucobuccal fold above the 2nd molar. Insert a 25-ga needle (bevel towards the bone) at the superior aspect of the mucobuccal fold above the 2nd molar.
- Remain at a 45 degree angle from the axis of the molars.
- Advance the needle for 2mm to 3mm superiorly, medially, and posteriorly. If you come in contact with bone, withdraw the needle and redirect 1mm more laterally.
- At a depth of 2mm to 3mm inject 3cc of anesthetic. (FIG 38 - right handed clinician injecting left side; FIG 39 - right handed clinician injecting right side).

POSTERIOR SUPERIOR ALVEOLAR BLOCK

FIG 38

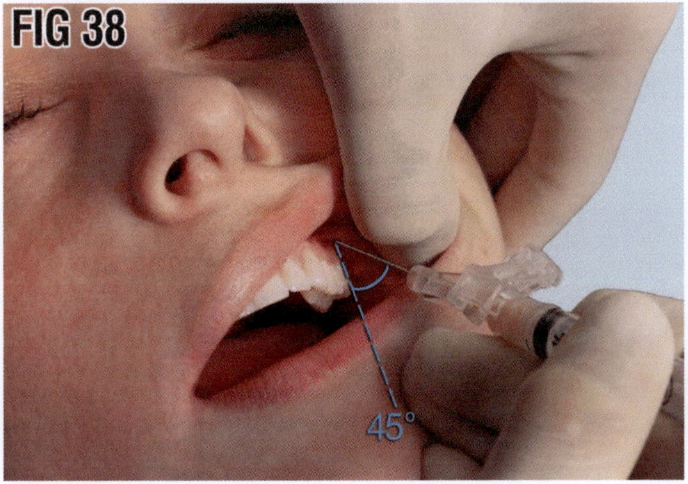

FIG 39

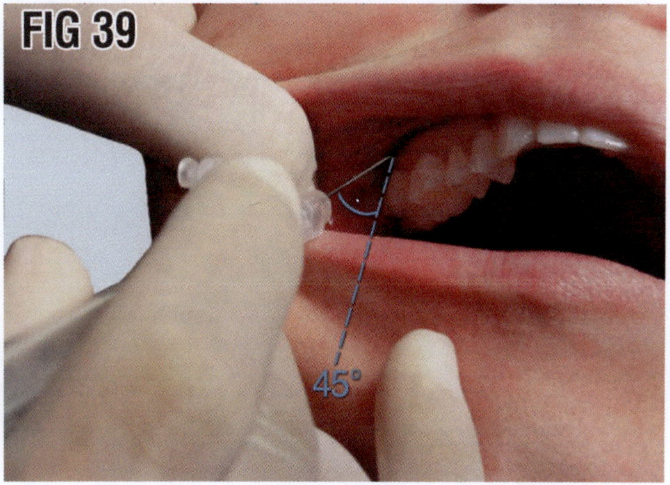

Sensory Distribution of the Inferior Alveolar Nerve:

Blocking the inferior alveolar nerve will provide anesthesia to the mandibular teeth, lower lip, and chin (FIG 40).

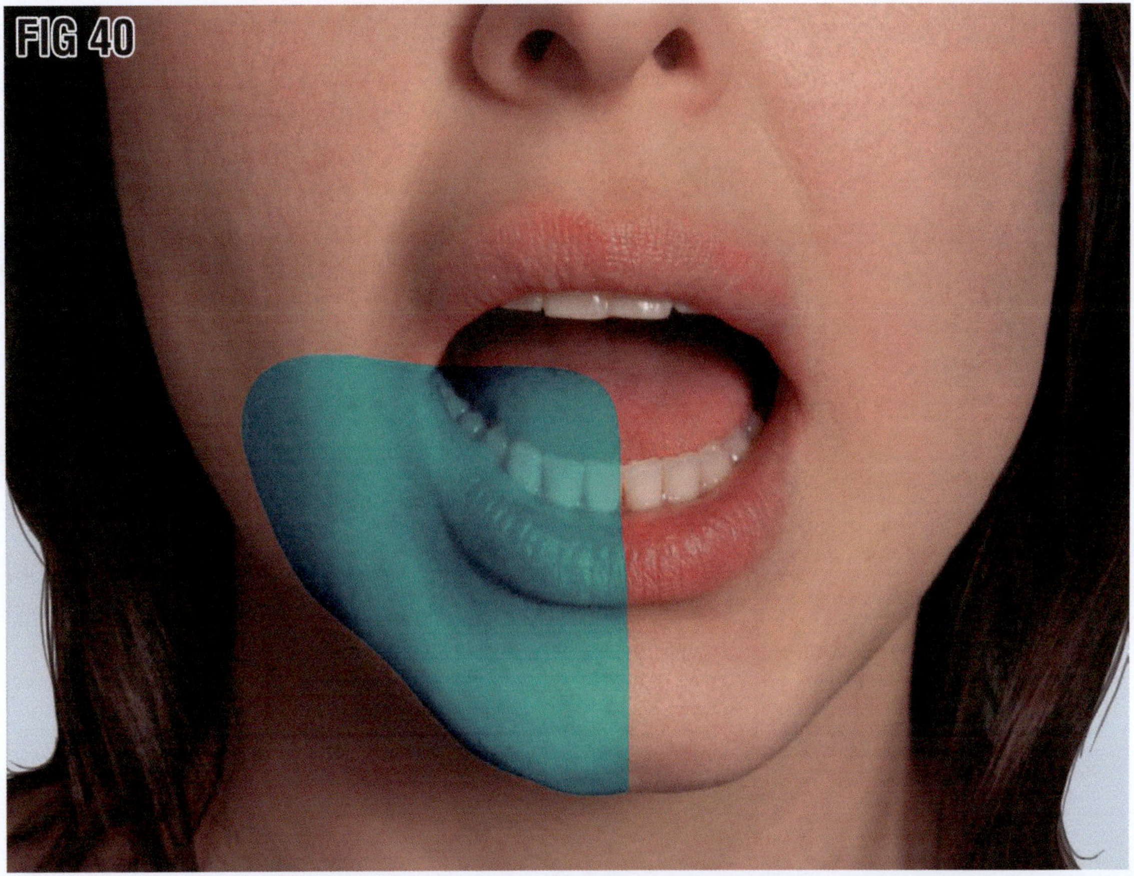
FIG 40

Inferior Alveolar Nerve Block (for mandibular molars):

- With the patient's mouth open, insert the non-dominant thumb into the mouth and rest its volar side against the buccal mucosa of the side receiving anesthesia. Make sure there is adequate light to see in the mouth.
- Pull the cheek laterally. With the non-dominant thumb inside the mouth and the other digits on the external surface of the cheek, grab onto the ramus of the mandible. The thumb on the inside should be positioned on the anterior surface of the ramus and the digits on the outside should be on the posterior surface of the ramus.
- Anesthetize the buccal mucosa with hurricane spray before injecting. Then insert the needle into the buccal mucosa at a 30 degree angle from the axis of the molars, away from the buccal mucosa. The point of entry should be 1cm above the occlusive surface of the posterior, inferior molar.
- Allow the needle to reach the bone, then pull back 2mm and inject 3cc of anesthetic (FIG 41 - right handed clinician injecting right side; FIG 42 - right handed clinician injecting left side).

Note: Depending on the side you are blocking and which is your dominant hand, you may have to cross over with the non-dominant hand in order to hold the mandible. While this may seem uncomfortable, I insist you hold the ramus with your non-dominant hand and the needle with your dominant hand for safety reasons.

INFERIOR ALVEOLAR NERVE BLOCK

FIG 41

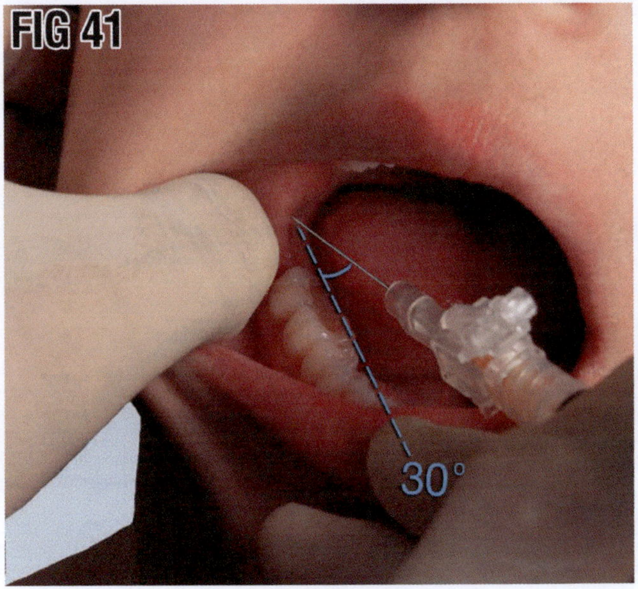

FIG 42

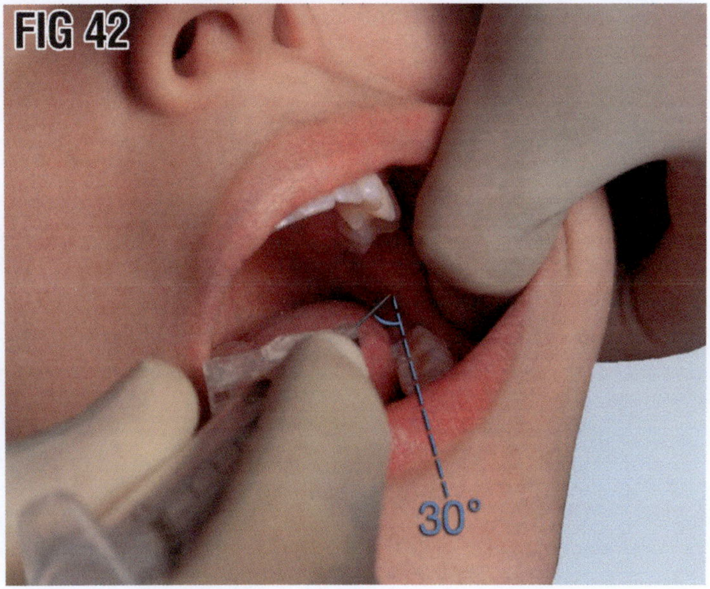

Sensory Distribution of Greater and Lesser Occipital Nerve:

Blocking the Greater and lesser Occipital nerves provides anesthesia to the occipital scalp for the respective side blocked. For the treatment of occipital neuralgia or tension headache, I recommend you block both sides.

Greater and Lesser Occipital Nerve Block:

- Palpate the superior aspect of mastoid process with your non-dominant hand on the side you are attempting to block. Then move medially and locate the external occipital protuberance.
- Locate the occipital artery between these two landmarks and aim just medial to the occipital artery. You should be at the level of the helix. That's the location of the greater occipital nerve.
- Insert a 25-ga needle at this point and advance the needle for about 2mm to 3mm.
- Inject 5cc of anesthetic.
- Block the lesser occipital nerve by moving 3.0 cm laterally and 1.0 cm inferiorly to the point just described.
- Insert here and inject another 5cc of anesthetic in a fan like distribution that covers this area (FIG 43).

Greater and Lesser Occipital Nerve Blocks with Epinephrine:

Since the scalp is the most vascularized skin surface of the human body, I suggest using epinephrine with lidocaine or bupivacaine when this block is attempted.

OCCIPITAL NERVE BLOCK

FIG 43

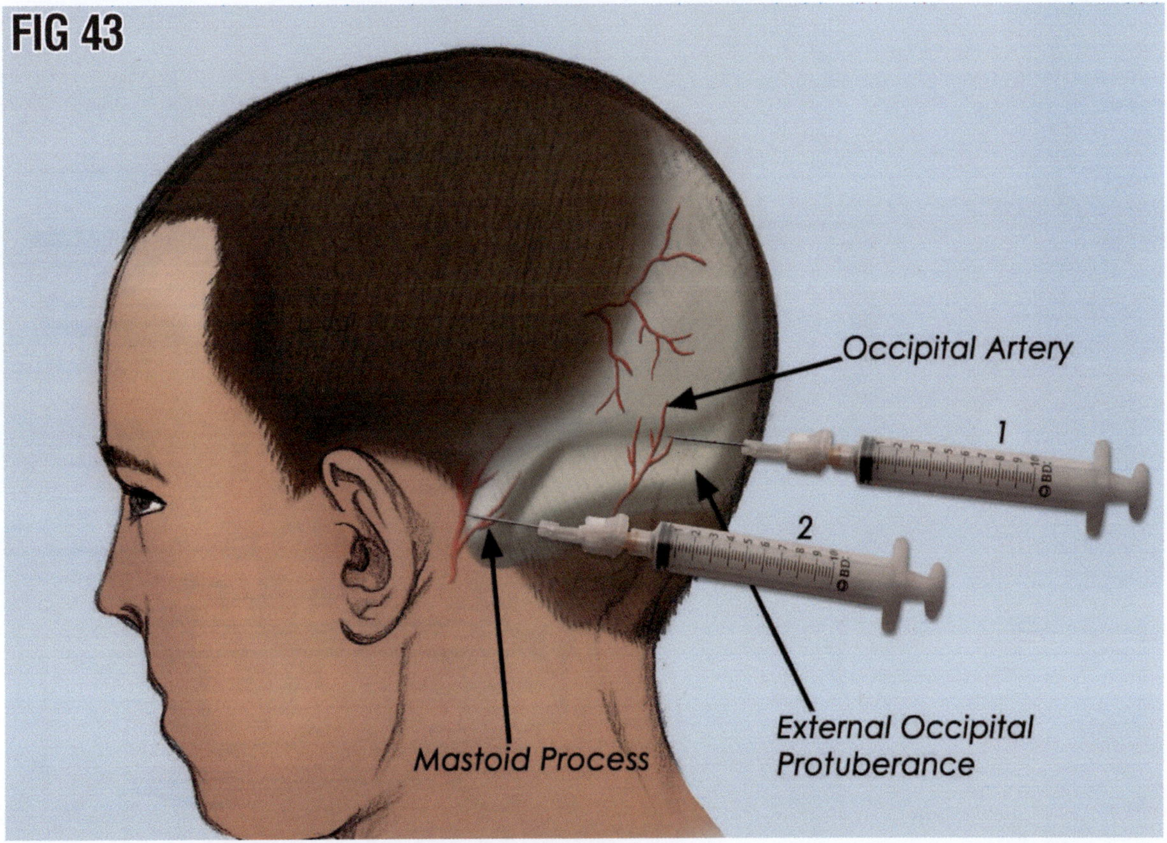

ADVANCED BLOCKS

Sensory Distribution of the Femoral Nerve:

Blocking the femoral nerve will provide anesthesia to the anterior thigh, the femur, and the knee.

Why do a femoral nerve block?

This is an advanced peripheral nerve block but I've included it in this manual because it is a useful block to alleviate femoral fracture pain. Also, I believe emergency medicine physicians are experts at identifying the correct landmarks for this particular block. We are well trained to place central lines in the femoral vein. In fact, EM physicians are known for placing these lines during codes and other time crunches when immediate central access is required. We find femoral veins quickly and with great accuracy. I believe we can find the femoral nerve just as easily.

Femoral Nerve Block:

- First locate the femoral artery as you would when trying to place a central line in the groin. The femoral artery is palpated 1cm below the inguinal ligament halfway between the pubic symphysis and the anterior iliac crest.
- Use 0.5% bupivacaine for 6 to 8 hours of anesthesia.
- Insert a 25-ga needle 1cm lateral to the femoral artery (remember the vein is medial).
- Insert at an angle of 60 degrees and point the needle superiorly.
- Aspirate to make sure no artery or vein has been cannulated. Similar to the "pop" which is felt when performing a spinal tap, feel for the "pop" when the needle transverses the femoral nerve sheath.
- If the patient complains of any paresthesia this means you are pressing on the nerve and should withdraw about one or two millimeters. Then inject 15cc of anesthetic.
- Massage the nerve sheath distally over the skin to encourage the spread of anesthesia superiorly (FIG 44).

FEMORAL NERVE BLOCK

FIG 44

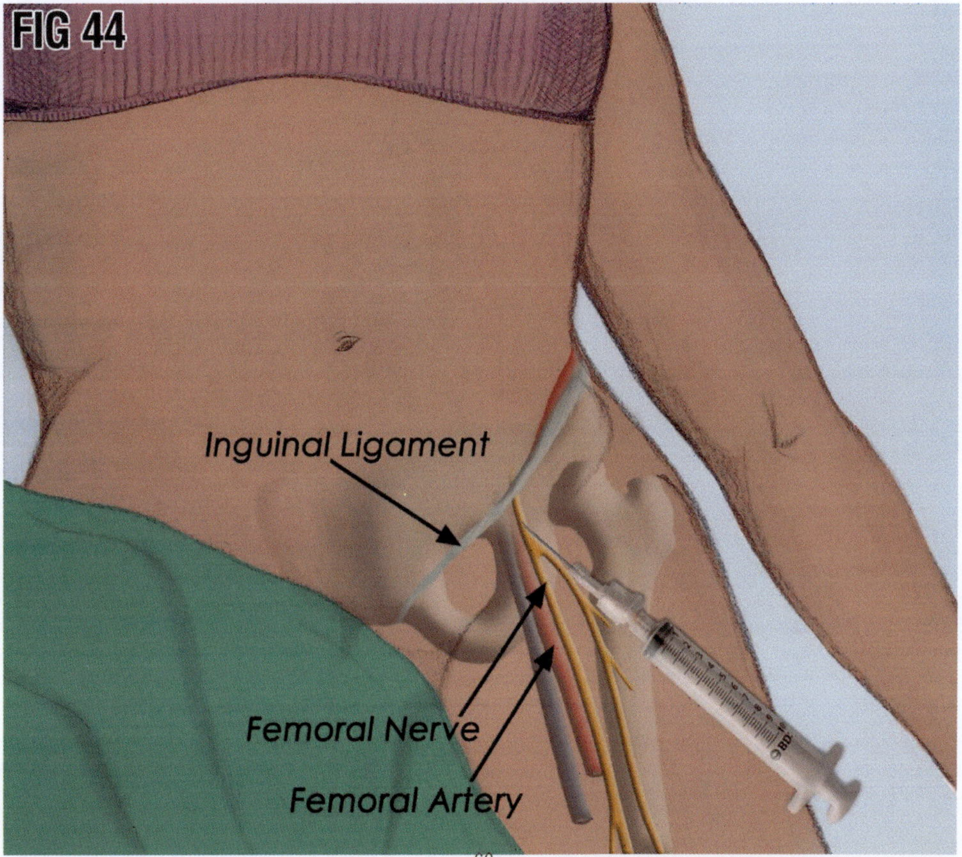

Sensory Distribution of Intercostal Nerves:

Blocking the intercostal nerve provides anesthesia over a band-like segment that extends from the lateral edge of the sternum to the vertebral spine.

Indications for an intercostal nerve block and some concerns:

The intercostal nerves are blocked to provide pain relief from rib fractures. If using bupivicaine with epinephrine the blocks can last up to 12 hours. The drawback is the reported 1.5% incidence of pneumothorax for each intercostal nerve blocked. This risk must be discussed with your patient and that discussion must be documented prior to attempting the procedure.

I have performed the intercostal block clinically when my patients have one painful rib fracture. I find the risk of pneumothorax too high if multiple ribs on the same side require anesthesia. Remember that one fractured rib will require the intercostal nerve block of that rib and at least one rib above and one rib below due to overlapping nerve fibers providing sensation. Multiple rib fractures require too many needle insertions in my opinion.

Intercostal Nerve Block:

- For the intercostal nerve receiving anesthesia retract the skin over that rib superiorly using the non-dominant index finger.
- With the skin retracted insert a 25-ga needle at the midpoint between the posterior axillary line and the vertebral spine. Maintain the needle 10 to 15 degrees off perpendicular with the needle tip pointing inferiorly.
- Advance to the lower border of the rib. At this point release the skin which puts the needle at the proper angle to advance further (FIG 45).
- Grab the syringe with the non-dominant hand and the shaft of the needle with the dominant hand (FIG 46). Now carefully walk the needle to the inferior edge of the rib by moving the shaft of the needle inferiorly with the dominant hand.
- Once at the edge of the rib advance the needle 3mm and inject 5cc of anesthetic (FIG 47). Repeat this inferior procedure one rib above and one rib below. Throughout, keep the palm of the hand holding the needle firmly in contact with the patient's body. This allows for best control.
- Keep in mind that the distance between the edge of the rib and the pleura is 8mm. Since you are advancing 3mm, you are getting relatively close to the pleura. That explains the 1.5% incidence of pneumothorax per intercostal block.

INTERCOSTAL NERVE BLOCK

FIG 45

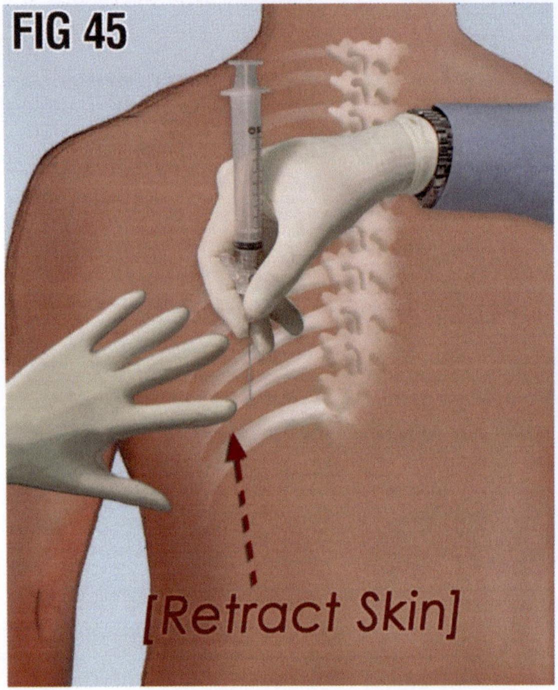

FIG 46

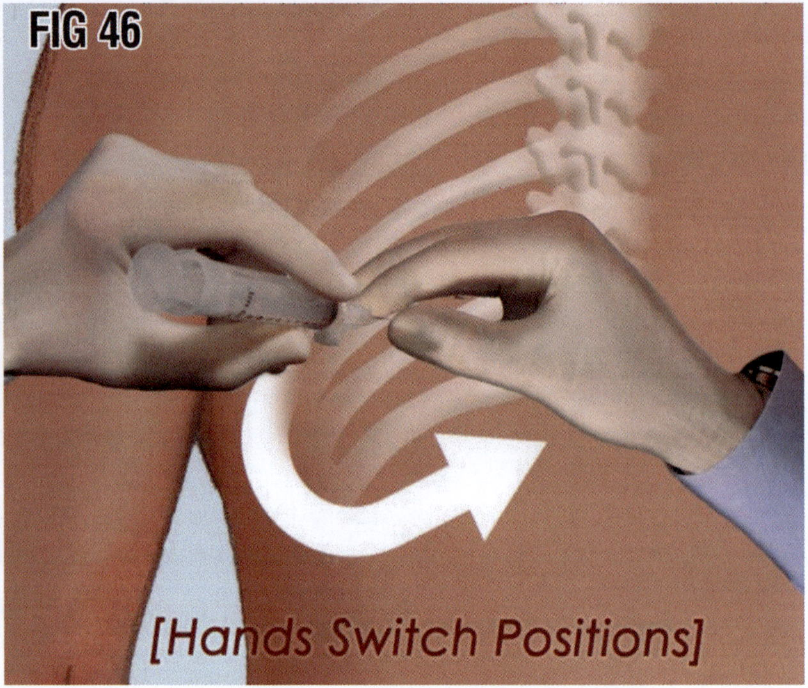

INTERCOSTAL NERVE BLOCK

FIG 47

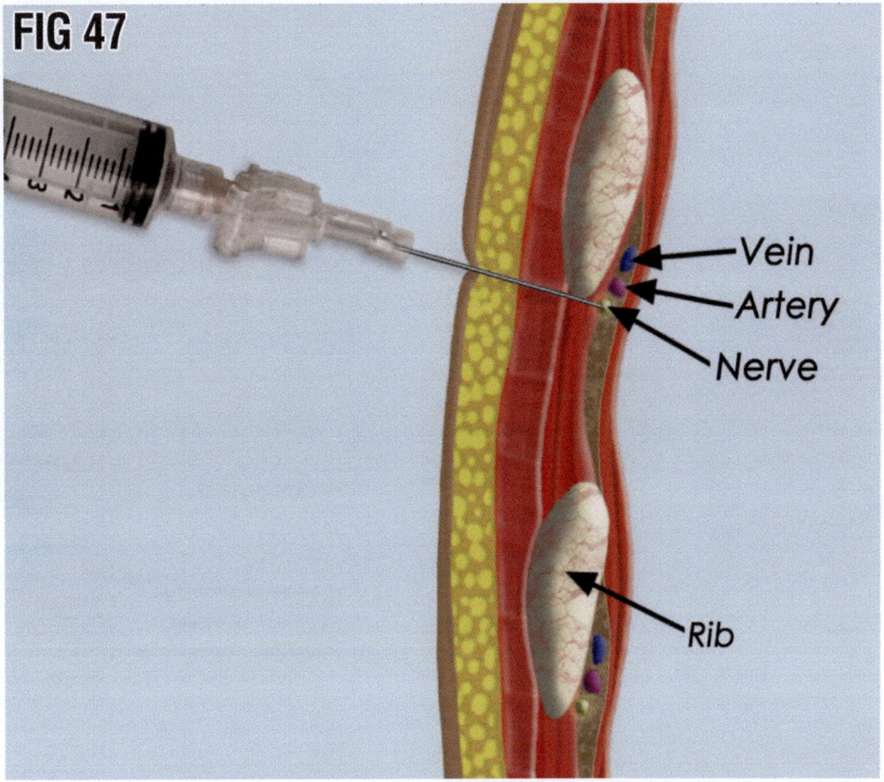

Penile Block:

I have performed a penile block two times in my career and in both cases the indication was a laceration repair to the penis itself.

Before attempting this block, study (FIG 48) (lateral view of the penis). Understand the boundaries of the triangular space delineated by the superficial fascia, the pubic symphysis and the corpus cavernosum.

Your plan is to provide anesthesia to the dorsal nerves of the penis by injecting in this triangular space on either side of the suspensory ligament. See (FIG 49).

PENILE NERVE BLOCK

FIG 48

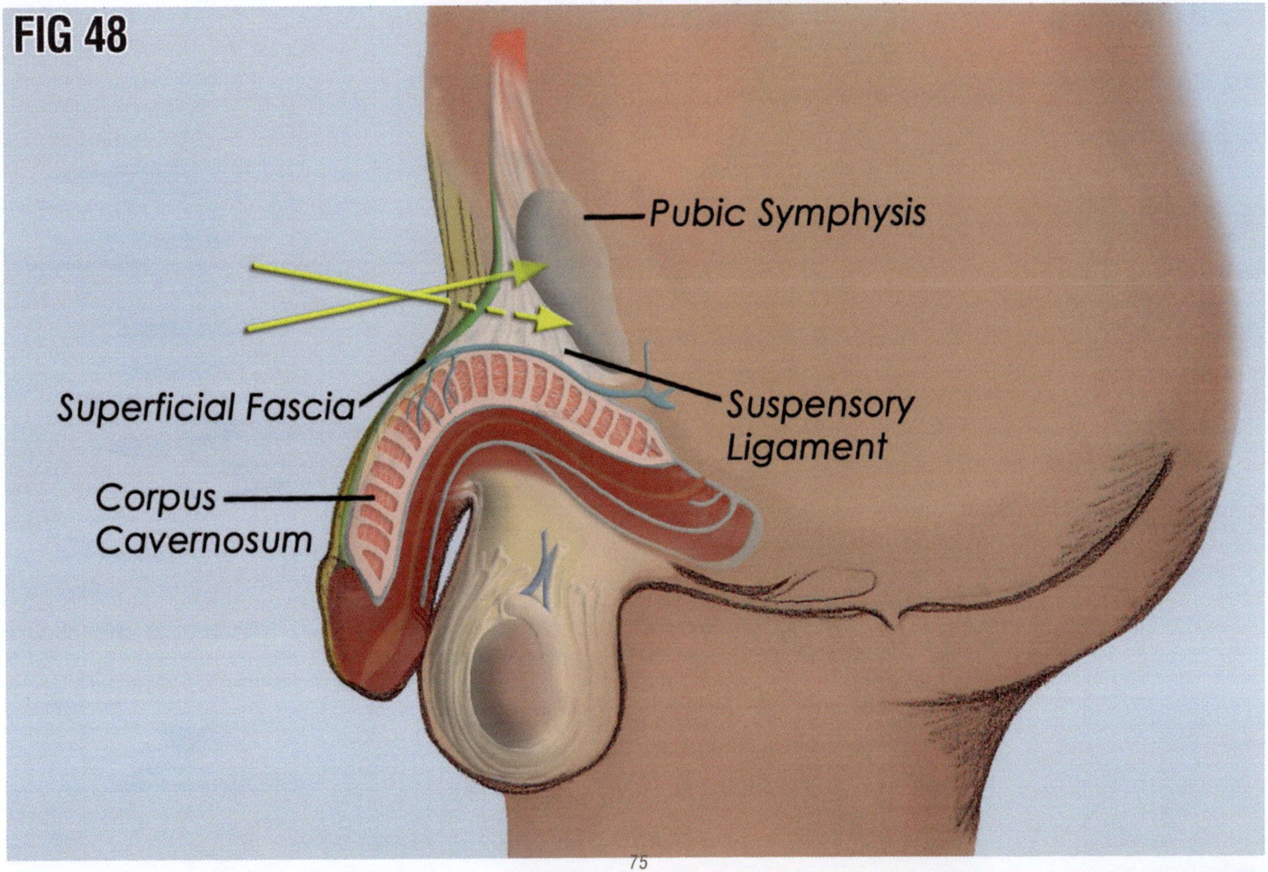

Blocking the Dorsal Nerve of the Penis:

- Make sure your patient is supine.
- Insert a 25-ga needle and advance it until it comes in contact with the pubic symphysis.
- Then withdraw the needle and redirect it 45 degrees from the midline and advance it under the pubic symphysis for 3-5 mm. Stay clear of the midline when advancing under the pubis.
- Inject 4cc of anesthetic at this point.
- Withdraw the needle and advance it at a 45 degree angle, for the same distance, on the other side.
- Inject an additional 4cc of anesthetic (FIG 48 & FIG 49).

PENILE NERVE BLOCK

FIG 49

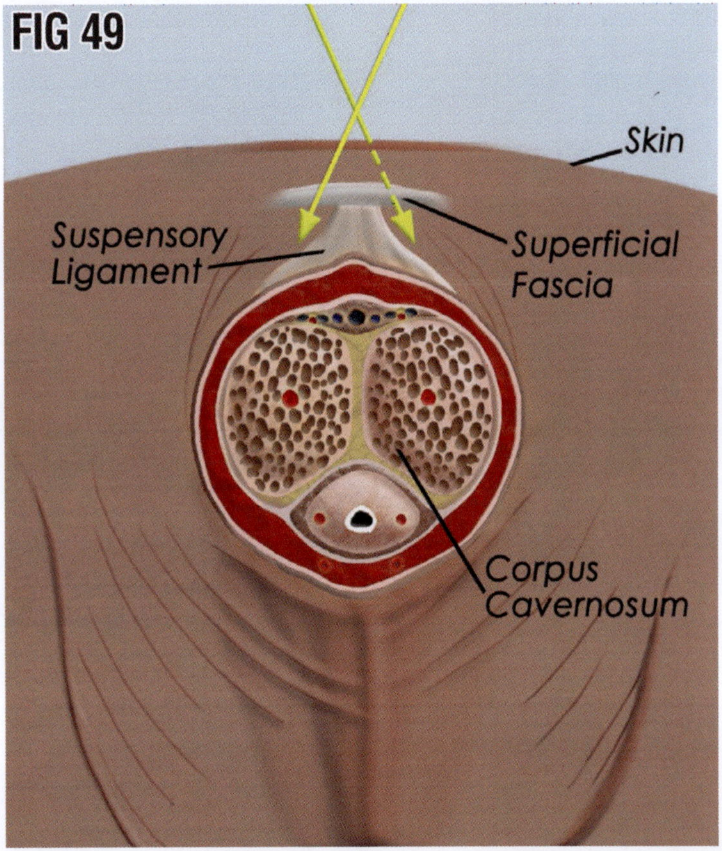

REFERENCES

Adriani J, Zepernick R, *Clinical effectiveness of drugs used for topical anesthesia.* JAMA, 188:93,1964.

Arthur DS, McNicol LR, *Local anesthetic techniques in paediatric surgery.* Br J Anesth, 58:760, 1986.

Bartfield JM, Gennis P, Barbera J, et al, *Buffered versus plain lidocaine as a local anesthetic for simple laceration repair.* Ann Emerg Med, 19: 1387, 1990.

Bovim G, Sand T, *Cervicogenic headache, migraine without aura and tension-type headache. Diagnostic blockade of greater occipital and supra-orbital nerves.* Pain, April; 53(1):111-2, 1993.

Chvapil M, Hameroff SR, O'Den K, et al, *Local anesthetics and wound healing,* J Surg Res, 27:367, 1979.

Covino BG: *Pharmacology of local anesthetic agents.* Br J Anaesth, 58:701, 1986.

Galindo A, *pH-adjusted local anesthetics, Clinical experience.* Reg Anesth, 8:35, 1983.

Kelly AM, Cohen M, Richards D, *Minimizing the pain of local infiltration anesthesia for wounds by injection into the wound edges.* J Emerg Med, 12:593, 1994.

Naja ZM, El Rajab M, *Occipital nerve blockade for cervicogenic headache: a double-blind randomized controlled clinical trial.* Pain Prac, Jun;6(2):89-95, 2006

Todd K, Berk WA, Huang R, *Effect of body locale and addition of epinephrine on the duration of action of a local anesthetic agent.* Ann Emerg Med, 21:723, 1992.

Pryor GJ, Kilpatrick WR, Opp DR, *Local anesthesia in minor lacerations: Topical TAC vs. lidocaine infiltration.* Ann Emerg Med, 9:568, 1980.

Printed in Dunstable, United Kingdom

91335485R00047